Injuries and Sports Medicine

Edited by Thomas Robert Wojda and Stanislaw P. Stawicki

Published in London, United Kingdom

Injuries and Sports Medicine
http://dx.doi.org/10.5772/intechopen.101015
Edited by Thomas Robert Wojda and Stanislaw P. Stawicki

Contributors
Merrick Wetzler, Ravin Patel, Austin Wetzler, Nicholas Bennett, Rodrigo Alonso Martínez Stenger, Heath P. Gould, Griffith G. George Gosnell, Brett A. Gerber, Gregory P. Guyton, Yusaku Sugiura, Yuji Takazawa, Kazuhiko Yamazaki, Kazuhiko Sakuma, Philip Shaheen, Eric Giza, Christopher Kreulen, Austin Lee

First published in London, United Kingdom, 2023 by IntechOpen
IntechOpen is the global imprint of INTECHOPEN LIMITED, registered in England and Wales, registration number: 11086078, 5 Princes Gate Court, London, SW7 2QJ, United Kingdom

British Library Cataloguing-in-Publication Data
A catalogue record for this book is available from the British Library

Additional hard and PDF copies can be obtained from orders@intechopen.com

Injuries and Sports Medicine
Edited by Thomas Robert Wojda and Stanislaw P. Stawicki
p. cm.
Print ISBN 978-1-80356-830-0
Online ISBN 978-1-80356-831-7
eBook (PDF) ISBN 978-1-80356-832-4

Meet the editors

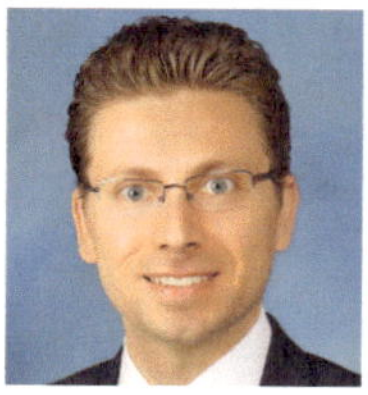

Dr. Thomas Robert Wojda graduated from the Medical University of Warsaw. He completed his Family Medicine residency at St. Luke's University Health Network in the Lehigh Valley, Pennsylvania, where he was also chief resident. During this time, he completed an MBA with a focus on leadership at the Ohio Dominican University, where he graduated *summa cum laude*. He then completed fellowships in sports medicine at Conemaugh Memorial Medical Center and University Orthopedics Center in Johnstown and Altoona, Pennsylvania, respectively. Currently, he is an Assistant Professor of Family Medicine at the University of Pittsburgh Medical Center (UPMC), a practicing primary care and sports medicine physician, and a fellow at the American College of Academic International Medicine.

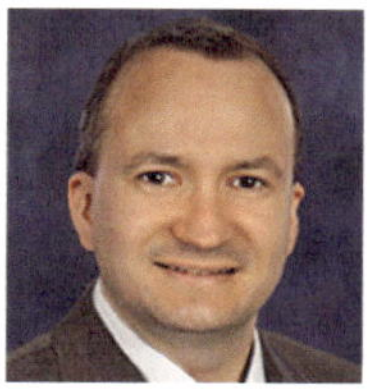

Dr. Stanislaw P. Stawicki is a Professor of Surgery and chair of the Department of Research and Innovation at St. Luke's University Health Network, Pennsylvania. A specialist in trauma, general surgery, and surgical critical care, he has co-authored more than 670 scholarly works, including more than 25 books. In addition to national and international medical leadership roles, Dr. Stawicki is a member of numerous editorial boards and grant evaluation/review bodies.

Contents

Preface

I have been involved in sports for as long as I can remember. I was always physically active growing up, pushed myself as far as I could go in soccer (football), was exposed to elite-level athletics, and played with and against players who would go on to ply their trade at a professional level. When I became a physician, I had the opportunity to amalgamate my love of sports and physical fitness with the discipline of medicine. As I have transitioned from competitive athletics to more recreational activity with a focus on health and wellness, I have witnessed the ubiquity of sports in our modern society. With an ageing population, there is a growing need for sports medicine to continue to evolve as more individuals are performing physical feats throughout their prolonged lifespan, incurring injuries as a consequence.

The growing rise of sports injuries and the need for evidence-based medicine in the treatment of various sport-related injuries have led to my editorship of this volume. I have worked in primary care, orthopedics, trauma surgery, and sports medicine. Each of these disciplines offers various levels of expertise as regards the diagnosis, prevention, treatment, and rehabilitation of sports-related injuries. As a medical provider who emphasizes the importance of physical fitness, over the years I have developed a keen sense of how to develop strong relationships with athletes to optimize their treatment regimens and enhance their performance. I am able to understand the stress these athletes' bodies endure, the pathophysiology behind various mechanical injuries, and the importance of the mental aspect of an athlete's road to recovery.

Sports medicine is a very intellectually thought-provoking field. As a former athlete, I enjoy the opportunity to be part of high-performing teams that sports medicine allows. The patients are often highly motivated, and other staff including trainers, physical therapists, coaches, and various other stakeholders all strive to achieve success together. On a more individual level, the ability to diagnose an ailment based on a well-taken history and thorough physical examination gives the medical provider a sense of satisfaction that they are alleviating suffering and improving patient care.

The chapters in this book reflect the expansion of sports medicine and its growing influence on healthcare. Production of the book would not have been possible without the contributions of the authors who are all experts in their respective fields of interest. I would like to thank Dr. Stanislaw Stawicki for his continued support throughout my academic medical journey. Lastly, I would like to thank the IntechOpen access community for providing scientifically curious minds with a platform to share and disseminate their work. I hope this book will aid all those who participate in sports and physical activity.

Thomas Robert Wojda
Assistant Professor,
Family Medicine,
University of Pittsburgh Medical Center (UPMC),
Pittsburgh, PA, USA

Stanislaw P. Stawicki
Professor of Surgery,
St. Luke's University Health Network,
Pennsylvania, USA

Chapter 1

Prevalent Orthopedic Injuries in Recreational Athletes after SARS-COV2 Lockdown: An Orthopedic Surgeon's Point of View in Order to Help Sport's Physicians Daily Practice

Rodrigo Alonso Martínez Stenger

Abstract

The conditions of compulsory social isolation in the course of 2020 due to severe acute respiratory syndrome coronavirus 2 (SARS-COV2) have forced even the most active individual to reduce their level of training and/or acquire sedentary habits. The effects of confinement have caused disarrangement, reflected in the loss of physical fitness because of lack of or decrease in training and changes in diet and healthy lifestyle. It has also caused modifications in psychosocial plane. This review analyzes the most frequently seen orthopedic injuries in recreational sports athletes after lockdown: muscle injuries, tendinopathies, acute or stress fractures, medial tibial stress syndrome, sprains, dislocations, and fasciitis.

Keywords: orthopedic injuries, risk factors, recreational athletes, lockdown

1. Introduction

Many recreational athletes who resumed their practice after a long period of detraining rejoined without noticing fatigue and discomfort, which precede the onset of pain. This situation, added to an incorrect periodization, graduation, and progression of workloads; inadequate nutrition and hydration; incorrect execution of the sports gesture with inappropriate movement patterns; and lack of rest and post-exercise recovery, generated a predisposition to suffer damage in some body tissues [1]. It should be noted that these situations occurred in stages prior to COVID-19 pandemic situation, but actually their prevalence has currently increased.

There are multiple variables that need to be addressed in order to recommend how to perform physical activities: type, frequency, intensity, duration, and density. There exist many guides related to this topic, but the special situation related to

COVID-19 generated high interest aimed to avoid injuries after an extended period of untraining [1].

The epidemiological analysis of sports injuries started with Dr. Roald Bahr's work. He described a methodological approach for the study of risk factors on sports injuries using Meeuwisse's multifactorial dynamic model in 2003 [2, 3]. Subsequently, several guidelines follow one another in terms of prevention strategies: from the linear cause-effect postulates of Quatman et al. [4] to the interactive models of Mendiguchia et al. [5] and complex systems, which have become widely known today with their "web of determinants" or "neural network" [6]. Broadly speaking, these works allow us to distinguish:

a. **Internal risk factors**, specific to each individual, which in turn are divided into nonmodifiable (age, anatomy, sex, previous injury, etc.) and modifiable (flexibility, dexterity, body composition, aerobic capacity, strength, neuromuscular control, etc.). They act as predisposers;

b. **External risk factors**, which correspond to characteristics of the external environment (playing field, footwear, equipment, etc.);

c. **Inciting event**, which can appear as a game situation, position of a joint in the surface on the ground, inappropriate movement pattern, collision, fall, etc.;

d. **Training load**, which is the stimulus applied to obtain an adaptive response. It must be prescribed appropriately because excessive workloads will produce fatigue and negative physiological effects as well as insufficient ones. On the other hand, appropriate stimuli will improve physical fitness, causing a positive physiological adaptation to the stress that it produces.

This is a dynamic process, since all these factors are interrelated and interact in multiple ways [6].

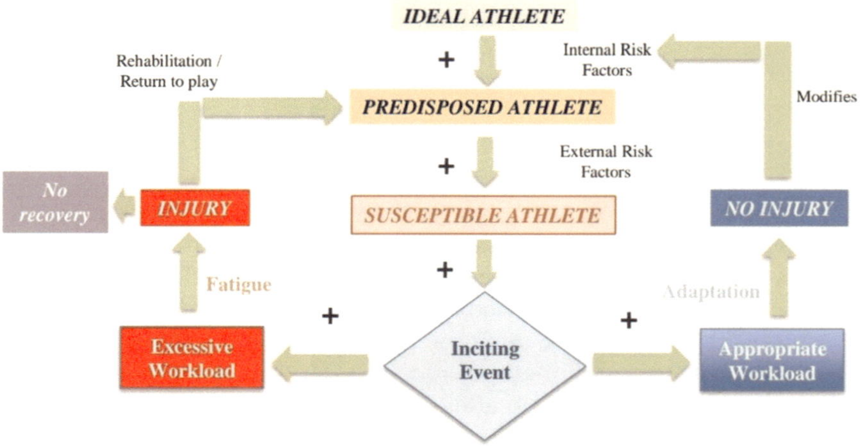

Figure 1.
Modified from "How do training and competition workloads relate to injury? The workload-injury etiology model."

Ideal athletes do not exist because they all have internal risk factors (**Figure 1**). The predisposed individual becomes susceptible when exposed to external risk factors. This fact, added to the application of a workload and the occurrence of an inciting event, can result in an adaptation to this stimulus or produce a failure/fatigue in the athlete's biopsychomechanics, with consequent damage to the different tissues of the anatomy and/or the psychic apparatus.

Excessive workload will cause an injury. Athletes can return to play with previous rehabilitation or not recover from this event.

Appropriate workload will generate adaptation, and this situation may modify internal risk factors.

Almost every injury is suffered as a devastating experience for an athlete. However, there is a large amount of evidence regarding the most effective treatment options for a particular type of injury in order to achieve an adequate return to play. It is important to note that there are many variables to have in mind when determining a treatment. Many of these factors have not been considered in the systematic reviews that were taken as a reference in this article, which represents an important area of research to be developed. These limitations, the quality of evidence and patient preferences, must be included when determining an appropriate treatment.

The analysis of epidemiological data is essential to identify risk factors, sport-specific patterns, and injury mechanisms, allowing to propose in this way prevention strategies that range from the introduction of protective equipment to changes in regulations and the field of play among other possible interventions in order to reduce the athlete's time out of training or competition. It will allow us to make effective decisions on preventive actions.

2. Muscle injuries

Muscle generates movement by contracting or relaxing. It makes up 40–45% of the total body mass. It is enveloped by fascia and attached to the skeleton by tendons. There are two types of muscle: striated (skeletal and cardiac) and smooth (found in the wall of hollow organs, for example). Its functional unit is the muscle fiber (or muscle cell), and there are two classes: red (type 1) and white (type 2) [7]. Type 1 fibers are slow-contracting fibers and resistant to fatigue, since they are located in postural muscles of the trunk (continuous activity). On the other hand, type 2 fibers are fast-contracting fibers, since they are located in upper and lower limbs.

Its functions include generating movement and mechanical energy (stored in glycogen), providing joint stability and protection to other deeper tissues, maintaining posture, and providing heat to the human body. It is an organ of greater adaptability since, being trainable, it can increase its strength and size [8]. It also has an endocrine function: acting on the brain (cognitive function), bone (mineralization), liver (carbohydrate metabolism), immune system (modulation), and adipose tissue (thermogenesis), among others [9].

Functional and structural muscle injuries [10] are produced by stretching too fast too far. Most of them are caused by noncontact situation: overload or overexertion [11]. They can also be generated by violent contraction against resistance or sudden uncoordinated and involuntary elongation. They are the most frequent injuries in athletes, and almost all of them occur at myotendinous junction [12]. It predominantly affects lower limbs (more frequently hamstrings). Modifiable risk factors can be identified: acceleration or deceleration movements, lack of warm-up and return to calm, muscle fatigue, large volume of training, and anabolic intake, among others. NOT modifiable risk factors include age older than 30 years, previous tear, biarticular muscles with type 2 fibers [13], etc. In order to diagnose muscle injuries, we recommend to start with a precise history of the occurrence, the circumstances, the symptoms, previous problems, followed by a careful clinical examination with inspection, palpation of the injured area, comparison to the other side, and testing of the function of the muscles. We will focus on structural muscle injuries in this review. There may be pain, functional disability or limitation (inability or decreased mobility of the affected area), local inflammation, hematoma, and sometimes audible "clicking." On certain occasions, when a frank muscular rupture occurs, a "gap" (defect similar to sinking) can be observed in the affected surface. It is important to establish a correlation of having made an exertion with the body segment involved. Some imaging studies must be carried out to verify the injury. Broadly speaking, trained sonographers will have no trouble identifying them. But it should be noted that this is an operator-dependent procedure. On certain occasions, a magnetic resonance imaging (MRI) will be required to reach an accurate diagnosis [14]. There are countless muscle injuries classifications, but currently the one described by FC Barcelona-Aspetar [15] presents the greatest advantages due to its detailed analysis regarding the type of injury and high-performance treatment strategy. It refers to the extracellular matrix involvement. For practical purposes, we will combine O'Donoghue [16] (symptoms-based) and Takebayashi et al. [17] (ultrasound-based) classification, which describes the following three types:

- Grade I: normal architecture, no appreciable tissue tear.
- Grade II: partial rupture of muscle fibers, with reduced strength of musculotendinous unit.
- Grade III: total rupture and complete loss of function.

Treatment will be conservative in grades I and II and will follow the premises of ***POLICE*** rule [18]. "**P**" represents ***Protection***. During the first 48 hours after the event occurred, the body weight will be unloaded (do not support the body segment involved). If lower limbs are affected, a pair of crutches may be used. "**OL**" implies starting gradually and progressively ***Optimal Loading***. Quick mobilization prevents hypertrophic scars and avoids reposterior ruptures; that is why patients should start loading if they are able to. "**I**" stands for ***Ice***, to be applied in periods of approximately 15–20 minutes, every 30 minutes. "**C**" refers to ***Compression***, which can be applied with an elastic bandage, thigh, calf, etc. "**E**" symbolizes ***Elevation*** of the affected limb in order to reduce edema and consequently pain.

Rehabilitation will be in charge of physiotherapists and involves sequential strengthening protocols according to pain tolerance and progressive evolution of patient's condition [15]. Regarding grade III injuries, surgical or conservative treatment will be considered according to age, functional limitation, affected region, occupation, activity level, etc. Complications consist of hypertrophic scars, fibrous nodules, myositis ossificans, and acute or stress compartment syndrome.

Prevention strategies include muscle eccentric training and strengthening, warm-up and cool-down practice, stretching, proprioception, correct technique, and avoiding muscle fatigue [15].

3. Tendinopathies

Tendons are connective tissue bands which insert muscle into bones. They transmit muscle contraction force to the bone in order to generate movement. Its relatively avascular structure implies a scarce regeneration process (producing nonelastic collagen fibers) if damage occurs [19]. Overuse causes repetitive microtrauma on the enthesis (insertion zone in the bone), exceeding self-intrinsic repair capacity [20]. It is important to highlight that these are NOT inflammatory changes. It produces local degenerative vascular and structural disorganization [21]. We also need to mention other causes of tendinopathy: rheumatological disorders (psoriasis, rheumatoid arthritis, etc.), metabolic diseases (gout, diabetes, hypercholesterolemia, etc.), and toxic (fluorinated) and pharmacological (statins) intake [22–25].

According to Blazina's classification, tendinopathies can cause pain at the end of sports practice (type I). It may start with the activity and disappear at the end of it (type II) or it could be permanent (type III). It can even cause tendon rupture (type IV). The most affected areas correspond to the medial and lateral elbow epicondyles (epicondylalgia), knee (patellar tendon), abdomen and pubis (groin pain—ex pubalgia), shoulder (subacromial compression syndrome—ex rotator cuff syndrome—most often affects supraspinatus muscle tendon), gluteal tendons, and the Achilles tendon.

Pain is the most important clinical feature. We can also identify local inflammation, decline in function or impotence, and reduced exercise tolerance. Sometimes, a clicking sound may occur if a rupture takes place. Tendinopathies develop gradually and progressively, although there may be cases of acute onset (especially type IV). Diagnosis is basically clinical, although images are sometimes required to rule out other associated injuries. Type I and II treatments consist of sports/work rest, after identifying the triggering-overloading repetitive action. Other alternative treatments include extracorporeal shock-wave therapy, nonsteroidal anti-inflammatory drug (NSAID) administration, kinesic therapies (Ciriax deep massage, eccentric exercises, etc.), platelet-rich plasma (PRP) injection, or 5% dextrose solution prolotherapy [26, 27]. Some type III injuries will be capable of nonsurgical treatments. In case it fails, tendinopathies will require surgery: longitudinal incisions, tenotomies, forage, or tendoscopy. Type IV injuries will be treated with tenorrhaphy or reinsertion.

4. Acute and stress fractures

Bone is a firm, hard, and resistant organ, which is part of vertebrate endoskeleton. It constitutes up to approximately 15% of the total body weight and is among the largest organs/systems of the human body [28]. Adult bone structure mainly includes cortical bone, cancellous bone (trabecular bone), and bone marrow cavity. Bone consists of three compartments: bone cells, extracellular organic matrix including collagen fibers and amorphous matrix, and extracellular minerals [29, 30]. There are three major types of cells in bone tissue: osteoblast (bone formation), osteoclast (bone resorption), and osteocytes (bone remodeling). Bone functions include supporting body movement, protection of internal organs, calcium storage, and blood cell production [29]. Recently, increasing studies have revealed that the skeleton contributes to whole body homeostasis and the maintenance of multiple important organs/systems, such as hematopoiesis, immune activity, energy metabolism, and brain function [31, 32].

Fracture is a loss of continuity in the cortical surface of the bone. Plastic deformity is more frequently seen in pediatric population since bone has a lower elasticity modulus. Fractures are produced by direct trauma (impact on the affected area), indirect trauma (at a distance from the region involved by transmission of forces), stress (repetitive microtraumas), or pre-existing pathologies (bone tumors, metastases, osteoporosis, etc.).

Symptoms include pain, local swelling, deformity or shortening, hematoma, functional limitation, or impotence. Sometimes, an audible click can take place. Exposed fractures show a skin wound in direct communication with the inside fracture site. Acute fractures have a clear traumatic history.

Stress fractures are produced by mechanical overuse in a prolonged period of time and account for 10% of all overuse sports injuries [33]. They will show progressive pain, without a clear onset. Bone tissue damage alternates with periods of remodeling, which causes a delay in the origin of symptoms. A complete cycle of bone turnover requires 3–4 months. When bone cannot remodel at the pace at which loading increases, it fractures [34]. Running is the most commonly associated sport—accounting for 69% of stress fractures [35]. Almost 95% occur in lower extremities due to the dissipation of ground reaction forces during load-bearing tasks such as marching, walking, running, or jumping [35]. Stress fractures typically occur in cortical bone in the following areas, in decreasing order of incidence: tibia, tarsal bones, metatarsals, femur, fibula, and pelvis [36, 37].

The diagnosis of acute fractures is made with simple frontal and profile radiographs (obliquely is demanded in distal regions: hands and feet). If there is a clear suspicion with a traumatic history and negative X-rays, sometimes computed tomography (CT) scan is requested. Periosteal reaction or continuity solution will be observed in one or both cortical surfaces. We can also use MRI, which will identify bone edema. Stress fractures will be diagnosed with these procedures or performing bone scintigraphy.

Treatment will be based on age, existence or not of bone exposure, affected bone, associated injuries, and functional demand of the patient, among other aspects. Broadly speaking, proximal and distal joint involving affected bone must be immobilized. ***POLICE*** rule will be applied according to tolerance. In other cases, surgical resolution will be chosen (reduction and osteosynthesis, osteodesis, arthroplasty, vertebroplasty, or arthrodesis, as appropriate). Exposed fracture constitutes a traumatic emergency and must be resolved in the operating room. Treatment will include washing and debridement of the wound, attempting to cover the exposure, stabilization of the fracture, antibiotic therapy, and tetanus prophylaxis. Stress fracture treatment should be analyzed in each particular case depending on the bone and affected area thereof, activity level of the patient, age, whether or not there is articular cartilage involvement, etc.

5. Medial tibial stress syndrome (MTSS)

Medial tibial stress syndrome is the most frequent overuse injury in runners and athletes involved in jumping. Incidences varying from 4–35% are reported, with both extremes being derived from military studies [38–40]. Clinically, it shows pain in posteromedial side of the mid- to distal tibia over a length of at least 5 cm during or some time after training [41, 42]. From the literature, it is unclear as to whether tibial stress fracture is a continuum of MTSS. In the 1970s, Roub et al. were the first to suggest that increased levels of stress to the tibia could result in a spectrum of bony overload. In this spectrum, the end stage was a cortical fracture. In the beginning of this spectrum, when bone resorption outpaces bone formation and replacement of the tibal cortex, MTSS occurs [43]. Differential diagnoses include nerve compressions, vascular pathologies, exertional compartment syndrome, and tibial stress fracture, among others [41]. Differentiation can usually be accomplished without additional imaging. Bone scintigraphy and magnetic resonance imaging (MRI) are widely used to confirm the diagnosis [44]. Treatment will follow ***POLICE*** rule guidelines. Rest and not supporting body weight is the most important advice.

6. Sprains

Ligaments are bands of elastic, fibrous connective tissue which hold bones together. Its function is to maintain "controlled mobility" of joints, giving passive stability, facilitating, and restricting certain actions. In addition, they give proprioceptive sensitivity to the involved joint. Sprain is considered a transitory loss of relations in an articular surface due to an overstretched ligament injury. Typically, a traumatic mechanism causes the ligament to stretch beyond its normal range, leading to injury. Ankle is the most frequently affected area in athletes.

Due to their clinical relevance in sports, we must mention knee injuries: anterior, posterior, lateral internal, and external cruciate ligament sprain or rupture, which can also be associated with meniscal injuries.

Ankle sprains manifest with pain, local inflammation, hematoma, impotence or functional limitation, clicking, feeling of instability, and intolerance to load. They are considered acute injuries. 78% of ankle sprains are caused by plantar inversion and flexion, a mechanism that usually affects the external lateral ligament (most frequently the anterior talofibular ligament).

Differential diagnosis should be made with other injuries that reproduce the same symptoms but are more serious, so radiographic images will be requested, thus excluding fractures and/or dislocations. On certain occasions, it will be necessary to request MRI to rule out soft tissue injuries: peroneal tendons, syndesmosis, deltoid ligament, etc. According to symptoms, we can classify sprains into three types: (1) mild, (2) moderate, and (3) severe. Type 1 is characterized by ligament elongation (sprain) without rupture, little or no functional limitation, mild edema, and joint pain and stability. In contrast, type 3 manifests with great functional impotence, hematoma, edema, pain, and instability due to total ligament rupture accompanied by joint capsule injury [45]. Treatment in mild grades of nonsports patients with stable ankle consists of applying ***POLICE*** rule for a 4–5-day period using a walker-type boot during 10 days, followed by gradual and progressive mobility according to tolerance for 2–3 weeks [46]. Currently, there is controversy regarding the treatment of type 3 sprains in high-performance athletes [45, 47]. Approximately 30% of ankle sprains are known to evolve into chronic instability, characterized by mobility greater than the functional limit, pain, edema and swelling, recurrent sprains, and the inability to perform physical activity. Treatment consists of performing proprioception exercises and strengthening peroneal muscles for a 6-week period. Faced with therapeutic failure, we proceed to surgical resolution.

7. Dislocations

Joints are areas where two or more bones join each other. They are classified into synarthrosis (immobile), amphiarthrosis (semimobile), and diarthrosis (mobile). In turn, diarthroses are subdivided into enarthrosis, condylarthrosis, troclearthrosis, reciprocal socket, trochoids, and arthrodesis. Dislocation is considered the loss of permanent contact of the articular surfaces, unlike sprain, which is characterized by being transitory. It can be caused by direct or indirect trauma. Clinically, pain, deformity, hematoma, edema, and inflammation associated with impotence or functional limitation can be observed. Diagnosis is established by X-ray (at least two projections: front and profile) where we will observe the "uncoupling" of involved bones. Associated injuries must also be ruled out. Treatment consists of performing reduction under anesthesia in the operating room. It constitutes an orthopedic emergency. Affected joint will be immobilized after evaluating post-reduction joint stability. In a second time, complementary studies may be requested to verify the indemnity or not of joint stabilizers. The most frequently affected joint in general population is the shoulder.

8. Fasciitis

Fascia is a connective tissue membrane that lines the muscles. In the plantar region, this structure is arranged from the base of the heel to the toes forming a wide band. Plantar fasciitis is the most common cause of heel pain, accounting for 80–90% of all cases. It is a chronic condition caused by traction on its insertion in the calcaneus bone. Sometimes, pain radiates toward the fingers. Its etiology remains unknown. Symptoms usually appear gradually and progressively after prolonged rest, can be established acutely, manifest during training, or be triggered by just walking or prolonged standing, in the most severe cases. A third part of all cases are bilateral. Plantar fasciitis is characterized by the exacerbation of pain on passive dorsiflexion of the fingers and forefoot, since this maneuver tightens the fascia. It can also be associated with morning stiffness. Diagnosis is made with the clinical examination. On certain occasions, images are needed both to rule out other pathologies and to confirm this condition. Treatment strategies include the use of NSAIDs, heel pads/insoles, night splints, and kinesic therapy based on stretching exercises and shock waves. In the case of nonsurgical treatment failure, open or arthroscopic fasciotomy will be performed.

9. Conclusions

Sports injuries lie in three fundamental aspects and their interrelationships: risk factors, inciting event, and work training load.

Gradual and progressive return to physical activity is recommended after a prolonged time of detraining in order to avoid injuries. Exercise must be performed in a structured and repetitive manner (at least at the beginning) through strength and/or resistance training.

Strength training should be performed using around 50% percent of maximum repetition (MR, three concentric and three eccentric with no rest in between). This planning produces the same benefits than training with 80% of MR (one concentric set, one eccentric set, and a rest set between them) and does not involve any specific equipment [48]. Exercises can be done with your own body weight, elastic bands, etc. Therefore, low-intensity and high-volume plans (lower loads and multiple repetitions) are preferred [49].

Resistance training must involve large muscle groups, such as jumping rope, jogging in place, burpees, and mountain climber.

Ideally, people can work in circuits doing quick repetition series, combining both strength and resistance training. It allows us to modify a number of circuits, series, and speed of execution [48].

Physical activity recommendation guidelines [50, 51] suggest 150–300 minutes per week of resistance training at moderate intensity (allows people to speak, but not sing) or vigorous (75–150 minutes per week, reaching that magnitude when only a few words can be told while performing training). Two or three muscle strength training sessions must be performed per week.

Coordination and balance should also be considered. Warm-up programs decrease injury rates by 30%. They include activities that increase body temperature and thus prepare tissues for maximum effort.

Static stretching exercises maintain body parts in a fixed position in order to relax certain muscles passively for at least 10–25 seconds. It improves flexibility and range of motion. Cooldown is also recommended when finishing.

If pain appears and/or remains (or even increases) in a period of 24 hours post-exercise, "too much too soon" could be the reason. Correct technique with proper movement patterns should always be executed before adding workload. A weekly increase in workload should not exceed 10%, since values above it contribute to injuries [52].

There is a better response to small increases (or decreases) in workload than to larger fluctuations on it.

Finally, you should have in mind that proper rest and recovery are essential part in training.

Author details

Rodrigo Alonso Martínez Stenger[1,2]

1 AMDARG (Argentinian Sport's Physicians Association) and Dr. A. Zubizarreta Hospital, Buenos Aires (Capital City), Argentina

2 World Skate Sport's Medicine Commission, Lausanne, Switzerland

*Address all correspondence to: rodrigomstenger@gmail.com

References

[1] Martínez Stenger R, Parrilla L, Khoury M. Cómo evitar el sedentarismo, la inactividad y limitar el riesgo de lesiones frente al retorno deportivo. Número 1 Revista AATD. 2020;**27**. Available from: https://www.google.com/url?sa=t&source=web&rct=j&url=https://revista.aatd.org.ar/wp-content/uploads/2020/12/REVISTA-AATD-2020-06-Como-evitar-el-sedentarismo.pdf&ved=2ahUKEwjR0ZPryaX4AhW6s5UCHXsEA2AQFnoECAgQAQ&usg=AOvVaw1WsAUcLJInfIMko-JfiRX0

[2] Meeuwisse W. Athletic injury etiology: Distinguishing between interaction and confounding. Clinical Journal of Sport Medicine. 1994;**4**:171-175

[3] Van Mechelen W, Hlobil H, Kemper C. Incidence, severity, aetiology and prevention of sports injuries. A review of concepts. Sports Medicine. 1992;**14**(2):82-99

[4] Quatman CE, Quatman CC, Hewett TE. Prediction and prevention of musculoskeletal injury: A paradigm shift in methodology. British Journal of Sports Medicine. Dec 2009;**43**(14):1100-1107

[5] Mendiguchia J, Alentorn-Geli E, Brughelli M. Hamstring strain injuries: Are we heading in the right direction? British Journal of Sports Medicine. 2012;**46**(2):81-85

[6] Bittencourt N, Meeuwisse W, Mendonça L, Nettel-Aguirre A, Ocarino J, Fonseca S. Complex systems approach for sports injuries: Moving from risk factor identification. British Journal of Sports Medicine. 2016;**50**(21):1309-1314

[7] Gillone C. Entrenamiento combinado de fuerza y resistencia. Ed. Panamericana. 2015. ISBN 9789500606677

[8] Schoepe T, Stelzer J, Garner D, Widrick J. Functional adaptability of muscle fibers to long-term resistance exercise. Medicine and Science in Sports and Exercise. 2003;**35**(6):944-951

[9] Christoph Hoffman, Cora Weigert. Skeletal muscle as an endocrine organ: The role of Myokines in exercise adaptations. Cold Spring Harbor Perspectives in Medicine. 2017;7(11):a029793

[10] Mueller-Wohlfahrt H-W, Haensel L, Mithoefer K, Ekstrand J, English B, McNally S, et al. Terminology and classification of muscle injuries in sports: The Munich consensus statement. British Journal of Sports Medicine. 2013;**47**(6):342-350

[11] Ekstrand J, Hagglund M, Walden M. Epidemiology of muscle injuries in professional football (soccer). The American Journal of Sports Medicine. 2011;**39**:1226-1232

[12] Jacobsen R, Krogsgaard M. The myotendinous junction – A vulnerable companion in sports: A narrative review. Frontiers in Physiology. 2021;**12**:635561

[13] Jarvinen T, Jarvinen L, Kaariainen M, et al. Muscle injuries: Biology & treatment. The American Journal of Sports Medicine. 2005;**33**:745-764

[14] Askling C, Tengvar M, Saartok T, et al. Acute fist-time hamstring strains during high speed running: A longitudinal study including clinical and magnetic resonance imaging findings. The American Journal of Sports Medicine. 2007;**35**:197-206

[15] FCBarcelona-Aspetar. Muscle injuries clinical guide 3.0. 2015

[16] O'Donoghue D. Treatment of Injuries to Athletes. Philadelphia, WB Saunders. 1962

[17] Takebayashi S, Takasawa H, Banzai Y, et al. Sonographic findings in muscle strain injury: Clinical and MR imaging correlation. Journal of Ultrasound in Medicine. 1995;**14**: 899-905

[18] Bahr y Maehlum. Lesiones deportivas. Diagnóstico, tratamiento y rehabilitación. Editorial Panamericana. 2007. ISBN 8498350069

[19] Lin TW, Cardenas L, Soslowsky LJ. Biomechanics of tendon injury and repair. Journal of Biomechanics. 2004;**37**: 865-877

[20] Magnusson SP, Langberg H, Kjaer M. The pathogenesis of tendinopathy: Balancing the response to loading. Nature Reviews Rheumatology. 2010;**6**:262-268

[21] Cook J, Purdam C. Is tendon pathology a continuum? A pathology model to explain the clinical presentation of load-induced tendinopathy. British Journal of Sports Medicine. 2009 Jun;**43** (6):409-416

[22] Scott A et al. Lipids, adiposity and tendinopathy: Is there a mechanistic link? Critical review. British Journal of Sports Medicine. 2015;**49**:984-988

[23] Abate M, Schiavone C, Salini V, Andia I. Occurrence of tendon pathologies in metabolic disorders. Rheumatology. 2013;**52**:599-608

[24] Ranger TA, Wong AM, Cook JL, Gaida JE. Is there an association between tendinopathy and diabetes mellitus? A systematic review with meta-analysis. British Journal of Sports Medicine. 2016; **50**:982-989

[25] Taylor B, Cheema A, Soslowsky L. Tendon pathology in hypercholesterolemia and familial hypercholesterolemia. Current Rheumatology Reports. 2017;**19**:76

[26] Brett M, Murrell G. Treatment of tendinopathy: What works, what does not, and what is on the horizon. Clinical Orthopaedics and Related Research. 2008;**466**(7):1539-1554

[27] FCBarcelona. Guía práctica clínica de las tendinopatías: diagnóstico, tratamiento y prevención. Apunts medicina de l'esport. 2012;**47**(176): 143-168. Available from: https://www.apunts.org/en-pdf-X0213371712807047

[28] Mizokami A, Kawakubo-Yasukochi T, Hirata M. Osteocalcin and its endocrine functions. Biochemical Pharmacology. 2017;**132**:1-8

[29] An YH, Martin KL. Handbook of Histology Methods for Bone and Cartilage. Totowa, USA: Humana Press; 2003. pp. 33-72

[30] Boskey AL, Posner AS. Bone structure, composition, and mineralization. The Orthopedic clinics of North America. 1984;**15**:597-612

[31] Asada N, Sato M, Katayama Y. Communication of bone cells with hematopoiesis, immunity and energy metabolism. BoneKEy Reports. 2015;**4**: 748

[32] Han Y, You X, Xing W, Zhang Z, Zou W. Paracrine and endocrine actions of bone-the functions of secretory proteins from osteoblasts, osteocytes, and osteoclasts. Bone Research. 2018;**6**:16

[33] McInnis KC, Ramey LN. High-risk stress fractures: Diagnosis and management. PM & R : The Journal of Injury, Function, and Rehabilitation. 2016;**8**:S113-S124

[34] Kohrt WM, Bloomfield SA, Little KD, Nelson ME, Yingling VR. ACSM position stand: Physical activity and bone health. Medicine and Science in Sports and Exercise. 2004;**36**: 1985-1996

[35] Miller TL, Best TM. Taking a holistic approach to managing difficult stress fractures. Journal of Orthopaedic Surgery and Research. 2016;**11**:98

[36] Matcuk GR, Mahanty SR, Skalski MR, et al. Stress fractures: Pathophysiology, clinical presentation, imaging features, and treatment options. Emergency Radiology. 2016;**23**: 365-375

[37] Mayer SW, Joyner PW, Almekinders LC, Parekh SG. Stress fractures of the foot and ankle in athletes. Sports Health. 2014;**6**(6): 481-489

[38] Andrish JT, Bergfeld JA, Walheim J. A prospective study on the management of shin splints. The Journal of Bone and Joint Surgery. American Volume. 1974; **56A**(8):1697-1700

[39] Bennett JE, Reinking MF, Pluemer B, et al. Factors contributing to the development of medial tibial stress syndrome in high school runners. Orthop Sports Phys Ther. 2001;**31**(9): 504-510

[40] Yates B, White S. The incidence and risk factors in the development of medial tibial stress syndrome among naval recruits. The American Journal of Sports Medicine. 2004;**32**(3):772-780

[41] American Medical Association. Standard Nomenclature of Athletic Injuries Presented by Subcommittee on Classification of Sports Injuries. Chicago (IL): AMA; 1966. p. 122

[42] Yates B, White S. The incidence and risk factors in the development of medial tibial stress syndrome among naval recruits. The American Journal of Sports Medicine. 2004;**32**(3):772-780

[43] Maarten H, Johannes L, Weir A, et al. Medial tibial stress syndrome: A critical review. Sports Medicine. 2009; **39**(7):523-546

[44] Boden BP, Osbahr DC, Jimenez C. Low-risk stress fractures. The American Journal of Sports Medicine. 2001;**29**(1): 100-111

[45] D'Hooghe P, Alkhelaifi K, et al. From "low" to "high" athletic ankle sprains: A comprehensive review. Operative Tech niques in Orthopaedics. 2018;**28**(2): 54-60

[46] D'Hooghe P, Cruz F, Alkhelaifi K. Return to play after a lateral ligament ankle sprain. Current Reviews in Musculoskeletal Medicine. 2020;**13**(3): 281-228

[47] Calder J, Bamford R, Petrie A, McCollum G. Stable versus unstable grade II high ankle sprains: A prospective study predicting the need for surgical stabilization and time to return to sports. Arthroscopy. 2016; **32**(4):634-642

[48] Muñoz-Martinez F, Rubi-Arias JA, Ramos-Campo D, Alcaraz P. Effectiveness of resistance circuit-based training for maximum oxygen uptake and upper-body one-repetition maximum improvements: A systematic review and meta-analysis. Sports Medicine. 2017;**47**(12):2553-2568

[49] Blackwell J, Atherton P, Smith K, Doleman B, Williams J, Lund J, et al. The efficacy of unsupervised home-based exercise regimens in comparison to

supervised laboratory-based exercise training upon cardio-respiratory health facets. Physiological Reports. 2017;**5**(17). Available from: https://pubmed.ncbi.nlm.nih.gov/28912129/

[50] Fiona C Bull, Salih S Al-Ansari, Stuart Biddle, Katja Borodulin, Matthew P Buman, Greet Cardon, et al. World Health Organization 2020 guidelines on physical activity and sedentary behaviour. British Journal of Sports Medicine. 2020;54(24):1451-1462.

[51] Piercy KL, Troiano RP, Ballard RM, Carlson SA, Fulton JE, Galuska DA, et al. The physical activity guidelines for Americans. JAMA. 2018;**320**(19): 2020-2028

[52] Harrison P, Johnston R. Relationship between training load, fitness & injury over an Australian rules football preseason. Journal of strength & conditioning research. 2017;**31**(10): 2686-2693

Chapter 2

Strategic Prevention Program of Hamstring Injuries in Sprinters

Yusaku Sugiura, Yuji Takazawa, Kazuhiko Yamazaki and Kazuhiko Sakuma

Abstract

Enhancing the functionality of the hamstring is an important matter for sprinters in improving their performance. Sprinters show almost the highest incidences of hamstring injuries as compared with other athletes. For sprinters and their coaches, prevention of hamstring injury is a prime concern along with improved their performance. To prevent hamstring injuries in sprinters, injury, incidence, mechanisms, and risk factors need to be taken into consideration, and a strategic program based on evidence needs to be implemented. A combination of three factors: agility, strength, and flexibility, is a good contributor to preventing muscle injuries in sprinters. Simultaneously, the training programs need to take into consideration the conditioning for muscle fatigue depending on a sprinter's abilities. It may be important for coaches, trainers, and sports doctors to encourage sprinters for stopping training to monitor the degree of fatigue objectively and subjectively and to avoid the risk of injury. Future establishment of a hamstring injury-prevention program will be achieved by building a support system for programs with tactics and strategies. These programs are based on the accumulation of data via cooperation among coaches, researchers, trainers, and sports doctors.

Keywords: hamstring injury, prevention program, sprinters

1. Introduction

In maximal sprinting, stride frequency plays a more decisive role than stride length does [1]. In addition, the large negative power for eccentric contraction of knee flexors (hamstrings) and the large positive power for concentric contraction of hip extensors contribute to high stride frequency, enabling the sprinter to run at higher speeds [2, 3]. Therefore, enhancing the functionality of the hamstrings is important to improve the performance of sprinters [2–4].

Sprinters nearly have the highest incidences of hamstring injuries compared with other athletes [5]. For sprinters and their coaches, the prevention of hamstring injuries is a primary concern alongside improving performance. However, clarifying the causal relationship between the cause and occurrence for hamstring injuries is challenging, as well as accumulating evidence for preventing hamstring injuries [6].

To prevent hamstring injuries in sprinters, injuries, incidences, mechanisms, and risk factors should be considered, and a strategic program based on evidence should

 IntechOpen

be implemented. The construction of modified prevention systems and the use of the latest technology will reduce hamstring injuries in sprinters. This contributes to the improvement of their performance.

2. Structure of the hamstrings

The hamstring muscle group consists of three major muscles of the posterior thigh, namely the semitendinosus, semimembranosus, and biceps femoris (long and short head) [7–9]. The long head of the biceps femoris, semitendinosus, and semimembranosus have a biarticular formation where they cross the knee and hip joints. The short head of the biceps femoris arises from the femur and inserts at the fibula head, making it a uniarticular muscle that crosses only the knee joint (**Figure 1**) [7–9].

Regarding the long head of the biceps femoris, the medial part of the ischial tuberosity represents the origin of the proximal tendon, while the distal insertion is on the lateral surface of the fibula head [7–9]. The semitendinosus has the same origin as the previous muscle; however, it is inserted on the medial tibial surface [7–9]. The proximal tendon of semimembranosus also has the same origin but originates from the lateral part, and the posterior aspect of the medial tibial condyle represents the distal insertion of the muscle [7–9].

The biceps femoris is the only component of the hamstring muscle group with dual innervation. The long head of the biceps femoris, semimembranosus, and semitendinosus are all innervated by the tibial branch of the sciatic nerve. The short head of the biceps femoris is innervated by the peroneal portion of the sciatic nerve.

Thus, the biceps femoris is considered a "hybrid" muscle [10] that has two heads with different origins and dual innervation. This feature may be a predisposing factor for hamstring injuries [11]. In research for elite track and field athletes in the British Athletics World Class [12], an isolated injury to the long head of biceps femoris was the most frequently occurring hamstring muscle injury (70%). Most injuries

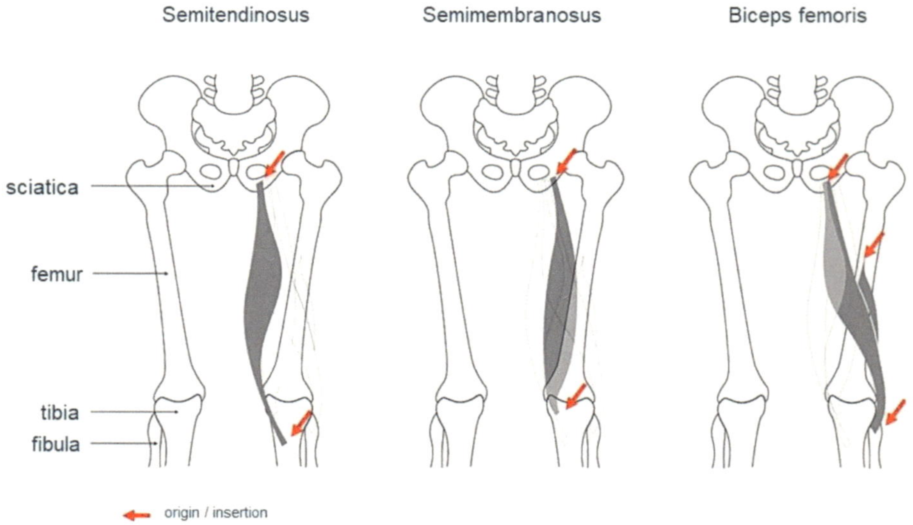

Figure 1.
Structure of the hamstrings.

occurred in the distal third of the hamstring (43%), with 31% in the proximal third and 26% in the central third.

The British Athletics Muscle Injury Classification is a reliable MRI-based classification system that categorizes the patients according to the injury site: myofascial (class a), muscle-tendon junction (class b) or intratendon injury (class c), and a numerical grading system (0–4) based on the extent of injury [13].

The isolated function of the hamstrings is to generate knee flexion and hip extension. During more integrated or dynamic muscle actions such as the stretch-shortening cycle [14–16] on sprinting, the hamstrings help in stabilizing the lumbopelvic hip complex and the knee joints [17, 18]. As such, hamstrings have unique structures (anatomy) and functions (physiology).

3. Biomechanics of high-speed running regarding hamstring injuries

A complete running cycle, that is, symmetrical and linear movement [19] in a sprinter includes two main phases: the contact phase in which the foot is in contact with the ground and the swing phase in which the foot is not in contact with the ground. Two main phases can be further divided into subphases: early contact (braking), late contact (population), early swing (thigh forward), and late swing (thigh back) (**Figure 2**) [19, 20].

In sprinters, hamstring injuries occur during high speed running, most likely because of the hamstrings along with its complex actions. The mechanism underlying this is attributed to its feature of being a biarticular muscle [14, 21], and its double innervation [22] works very rapidly to generate a large amount of power.

As hamstrings muscles are mainly hip extensors, they work in the late swing phase of sprinting to concentrically and quickly get the thigh back [2, 4] while acting as knee flexors to eccentrically decelerate the forward swing of the lower leg [2, 4, 14]. In the early contact phase, the hamstrings apply concentric action as knee flexor and hip extensor muscles to reduce the loss in running speed, which shifts the body's center of gravity forward smoothly [14, 23]. To maximize running speed during sprinting, the hamstrings must generate a large amount of power in these phases [2, 3, 24].

From the late swing phase to the early contact phase during full-speed running, the hamstrings must rapidly switch from eccentric contractions to concentric

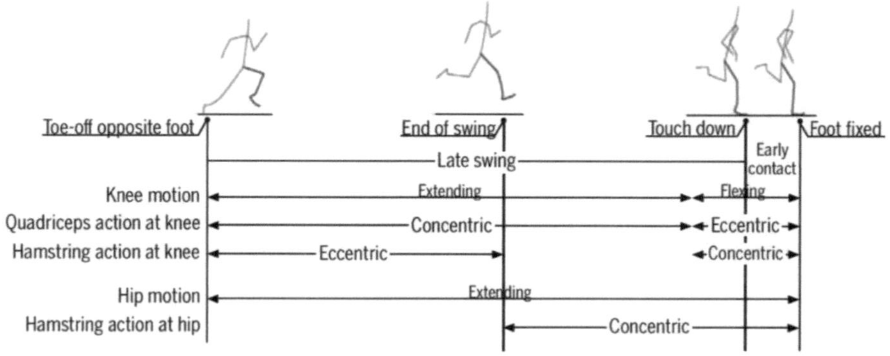

Figure 2.
Dominant quadriceps and hamstring contraction modes (the muscle contractions are concentric and eccentric) in the late swing and early contact phases of sprinting [19].

contractions (stretch-shortening cycle) [14–16] while under the influence of the contractile activity of the quadriceps femoris muscle [25]. These actions generate high forces, which have been postulated to be related to hamstring injuries [15], are commonly seen in sprinters [26, 27].

Most researchers investigating the role of the hamstring during sprint argue that the late swing phase is likely to be the point in the running cycle at which the hamstrings are most susceptible to injuries [18, 28–32]. A few researchers speculated that the early contact phase would be the highest risk point of sprint [4, 24]. Most of the injuries occur during the late swing and early contact phases of running.

4. Presenting risk factors regarding hamstring injuries

In 1985, Agre [33] discussed hamstring injuries occurring while running or sprinting. He listed several possible factors related to hamstring injuries, which are widely accepted in the research and clinical fields; they include (1) inadequacy of muscle flexibility, (2) muscle strength and/or endurance, and (3) warm-up and stretching before activity; (4) dys-synergic muscle contraction; (5) awkward running style; and (6) resumption of activity before complete rehabilitation.

In a theoretical model, Worrell [34] suggests that the increase in the risk of hamstring injuries is because of a mix of abnormalities related to strength, flexibility, warm-up method, and fatigue. Devlin [35] posits a threshold above which the number of risk factors contributes to injuries. Therefore, some factors are potentially more capable of predicting injuries than others.

Based on the results of practical research conducted by Sugiura et al. [6], strength deficits, lack of neuromuscular control, and lack of flexibility contribute to the incidence of hamstring injuries. However, the effects of each of the three factors on hamstring injuries have not been examined. This chapter provides an overview of factors 1–3 (**Table 1**).

4.1 Inadequate muscle strength

Many studies have examined the causes of hamstring injuries related to leg muscle strength. Previous studies have emphasized the relationship between hamstring weakness during eccentric contraction and muscle injuries [15, 16, 36].

However, in 2008, Sugiura et al. [37] reported that muscle weakness during eccentric contraction of the hamstring (hip extensor) can also contribute to hamstring injuries. Whichever it is, insufficient hamstring strength, left-to-right muscle imbalance, and decreased hamstring strength relative to quadriceps strength (H/Q ratios) are thought to cause hamstring injuries.

Cause		**Result**
One and/or more of risk factor	Trigger	Onset
Inadequate muscle strength Ds-synergic muscle contraction Inadequate flexibility of muscles	High-speed running	Hamstring injuries

Table 1.
Cause and result for hamstring injuries.

Insufficient hamstring strength weakens the contraction force and causes the thigh back to swing quickly in late swing phase. Moreover, in the early contact phase, the hip joint extension torque could not be exerted sufficiently. This results in excessive eccentric load on the hamstrings, which was presumed to cause hamstring injuries.

4.2 Dys-synergic muscle contraction

Hamstrings are involved in leg movements in various sports events. Among them, in sprinting, which requires high speed, the hamstrings contribute significantly to performance compared with other events.

During sprinting, the hamstrings are not affected by the activity of the quadriceps femoris. Sprinters should respond rapidly from eccentric contraction to concentric contraction (stretch-shortening cycle) [14–16] from the late swing phase to the early contact phase. Sprinters exert more power in split second and achieve higher speeds by using the stretch-shortening cycle. Neuromuscular coordination plays an important role in these mechanisms. From the late swing phase to the early contact phase, if there is ataxia, such as changes in the contraction strength of the hamstring or dys-synergic muscle contraction, the hamstring injuries will become onset [33].

4.3 Inadequate flexibility of the muscles

As the flexibility of the hamstring decreases, the "knee flexion angle–torque relationship" shifts to the left (37). This indicates that the hamstring length at the peak torque is shorter. In the tension-length relationship of the muscles, shortening optimal for muscle length means that the resistance to the eccentric load is low. Brockett et al. [38] concluded that a shorter muscle length at peak torque is a risk factor for hamstring injuries.

Sprinting involves moving leg joints through a large range of motion as much power as possible. The lack of hamstring flexibility will lead to hamstring injuries.

5. How to prevent hamstring injuries

In ball sports, hamstring injuries occur when turning sharply or cutting [39], whereas in sprinting, injuries often occur while running at high speed [16, 33]. Two types of hamstring injuries, defined by the injury mechanism, have been described as stretch- and sprint-type hamstring injuries [40]. Stretch-type hamstring injuries occur on movements involving a combination of extreme hip flexion and knee extension such as kicking and maneuvers, whereas sprint-type hamstring injuries occur during maximal or near-maximal running movement [41]. Therefore, hamstring injury types on ball sports players are of stretch and sprint complex types.

To obtain useful information for a hamstring injury prevention program, it is desirable to conduct research on sprinters for track and field. A hamstring prevention program for sprinters could become a standard prescription for many events, including ball sports.

5.1 Onset of hamstring injuries related to hamstring weakness

The muscle strength of the hamstrings, hip extensor, and quadriceps was measured and related to the subsequent occurrence of hamstring injuries over a 1-year period of a prospective study [37]. Isokinetic testing was performed on 30 male elite sprinters for the assessment of hip extensors, quadriceps, and hamstring strength. The methods used for testing muscle strength simulate the specific muscle action during the late swing and early contact phases while sprinting. The strength of the hip extensors, quadriceps, and hamstrings, as well as the H/Q ratios, was compared between uninjured and injured sprinters.

During the research period, a hamstring injury in one lower limb occurred in six sprinters (10.0% of 60 lower extremities). All injuries were sustained while sprinting. The participants were divided into the uninjured group (comprised of 48 lower limbs in 24 participants) and injured group (comprised 12 lower limbs in six subjects).

At a speed of 60/s, the torque of the hamstrings measured eccentrically about the knee and concentrically about the hip was significantly lower for the injured lower limb than for the uninjured limb (**Figure 3**). The differences in H/Q ratios between the uninjured and injured lower limbs in the injured group were solely attributable to the differences in hamstring strength. These results suggest that the weakness of the hamstrings and possibly hip extensors is a cause of injuries (**Figure 4**).

The onset of hamstring injuries in elite sprinters was related to hamstring weakness during eccentric contractions across the knee and concentric contractions across the hip. The identification of sprinters with unilateral weakness of the hip extensors and knee flexors may reduce the incidence of hamstring injuries.

This study focused on the relationship between muscle strength and the occurrence of hamstring injuries. Other factors such as agility and flexibility may have contributed to the occurrence of hamstring injuries.

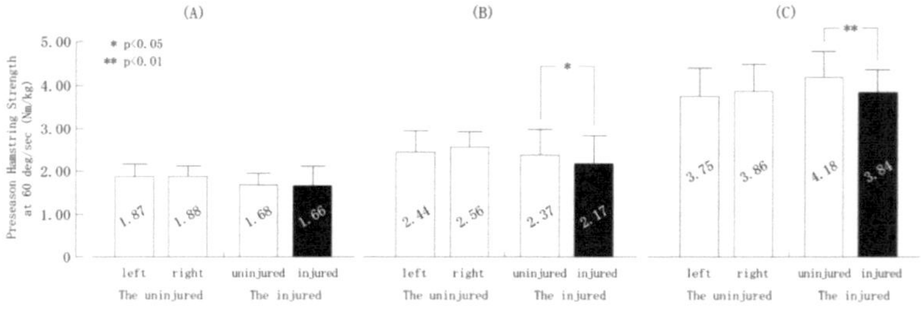

Figure 3.
Mean (SD) preseason hamstring strength for sprinters who did not experience the hamstring strain (the uninjured: n = 24) compared with sprinters who subsequently sustained the hamstring strain (the injured: n = 6). (A): Knee flexion-concentric (B): Knee flexion-eccentric (C): Hip extension-concentric.

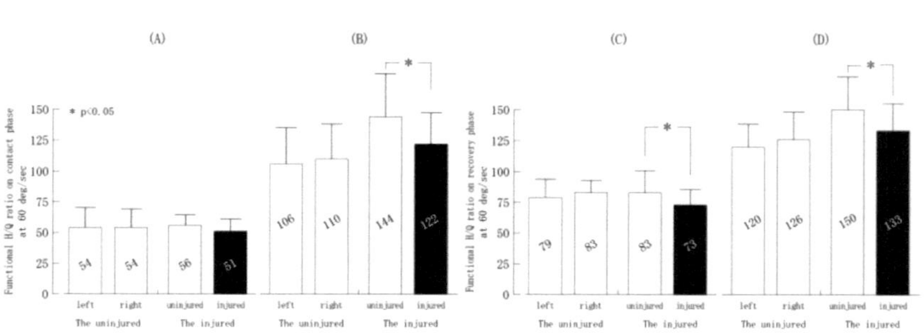

Figure 4.
Mean (SD) preseason functional H/Q on contact (A), (B) and recovery (C), (D) phase for sprinters who did not the hamstring strain (the uninjured: n = 24) compared with sprinters who subsequently sustained the hamstring strain (the injured: n = 6). (A): Knee flexion-concentric/knee extension-eccentric (B): Hip extension-concentric/knee extension-eccentric (C): Knee flexion-eccentric/knee extension-concentric (D): Hip extension-concentric/knee extension-concentric.

5.2 Effects of prevention program on hamstring injuries

A total of 613 collegiate male sprinters employed submaximal/maximal running for several runs and supramaximal running for a few runs throughout their 24 years of training [6, 19, 25]. The hamstring injury prevention program had become the most effective strategy in 24 years. The program was divided into three periods: period I that covered four seasons (1988–1991), period II that covered eight seasons (1992–1999), and period III that covered 12 seasons (2000–2011).

5.2.1 Strategic combination programs to prevent hamstring injuries

The injury prevention program for sprinters has evolved over time to reflect the current most effective strategies for preventing hamstring injuries (**Table 2**). New programs and equipment were developed and introduced for the Olympic Games of Seoul, Barcelona, and Sydney. As a result, the number of programs has increased and prevention programs evolved [6, 19, 25].

For an appropriate prevention program, the coach modified the program through trial and error while investigating causative factors. Consequently, the program aimed to improve neuromuscular function, muscle strength, and dynamic flexibility.

Period I only consisted of performing concentric hamstring strengthening with help of a traditional leg curl weight machine. Period II is similar to the period I program but with additional agility training, including ladder and mini-hurdle exercises. To allow a concentric hip extension exercise, a newly developed weight machine was introduced in the middle of period II. In period III, eccentric hamstring strengthening exercises (Nordic hamstring exercise [42, 43], glute-ham raise exercises, [44], and dynamic stretching exercises) were added in addition to the programs implemented in period II.

Objective and method	Action and/or Motion (Load)	Period		
		I	II	III
Strength				
Weight macine	Knee flexors concentrically (leg curl) (3/5–4/5 of body weight × 10 repetitions × 3–5 sets)	•	•	•
	Hip extensors concentrically (hip extension) (4/5–5/5 of body weight ×10 repetitions × 3–5 sets)		•	•
Body weight	Knee flexors eccentrically (Nordic hamstring exercise) (lean forward slowly × 30–60 seconds × 5 sets)			•
	Knee flexors eccentrically and hip extensors/knee flexors concentrically (glute-ham raise) (lean forward, downword, and upward × 10–20 repetitions × 5 sets)			•
Agility				
Ladder	5 types of fast stepping in all directions (10 m × 4 repetitions)		•	•
Mini-hurdle	4 types of one and/or both leg(s) with fast stepping (10 hurdles × 4 repetitions)		•	•
Flexibility				
Dynamic stretching	3 types of stretching for muscles around hip joint (20 m × 1 repetitiion)			•

Table 2.
Description of the standard preventive program for hamstring injuries.

The sprinters performed all program parts according to the loads, actions, and motions designated for each program, as mentioned in **Table 1**. In each case, the program used was modified according to the coach's judgment, considering the condition of the sprinter. Strength training was considered as a part of the weight training, and agility/flexibility training was performed during warm-ups.

5.2.2 Prescription for volume/quality of overall sprint training throughout the year

Figure 5 presents the standard program with usual and special training arranged for the overall sprint training applied throughout the year. Training program was divided into six phases: recovery, basic training, preseason, first season, interseason, and second season.

Excluding the recovery phase, the regular training for submaximal and maximum running was completed in five phases. In contrast, specialized training for supramaximal running was carried out within a short time, weeks, in four phases, eliminating the recovery and basic phases. With modifications to volume and quality, three types of running—submaximal, maximum, and supramaximal—were carried out throughout the year, except for the recovery phase.

5.2.3 Submaximal and maximal running for volume training

Submaximal and maximal running types are types of volume training (**Figure 5**). Submaximal and maximal running types have sufficient volume to cause overload,

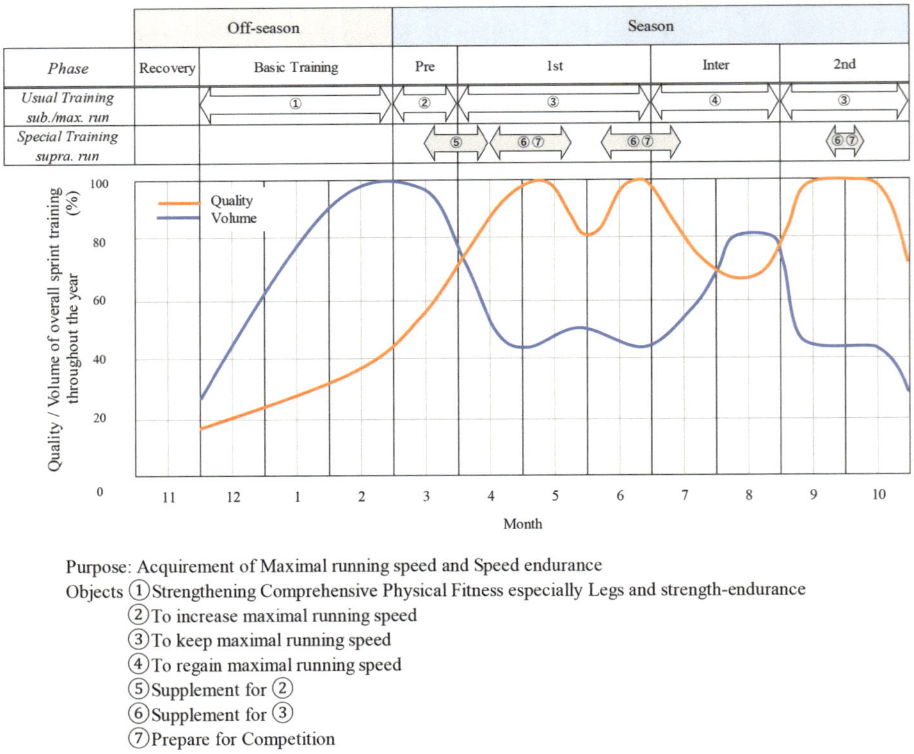

Figure 5.
Concepts of overall sprint training program throughout the year.

Training Contents	
BasicTraining:①	**Pre-season:②**
30 minutes build up every 10 minutes for Cross–Country 100 m at 70% OR 200 m at 60% 10–20 repetition for Up Hill Running 100–150 m 10 kg – Weights x 5 repetitions on Sled for Resistance Running. 200–300 m at 60% 10 repetitions 250–400 m at 60% 10 repetitions	50–100 m 10 kg–Weights x 5 repetitions on Sled for Resistance Running 150–200 m at 80–90% 3 repetition x 2–4 sets 300 m at 70–80% 5 repetitions 1–2 sets
1st and 2nd–season:③	Inter–season:④
50–100 m 5 kg–Weights x 2 repetitions on Sled for Resistance Running 30–60 m at 90–100% 5 repetitions for Start Dash and (100 m at 95%, 150 m at 95%, 200 m at 90%) 1–2 sets 30–60 m at 90–100% 5 repetitions for Start Dash and (100–120 m at 95%) 3–5 repetitions, 50 m at a constant tempo for Skip x 5 repetitions 30–60 m at 90–100% 5 repetitions for Start Dash and (200 mat 90%, 400 m at 90%) 1–2 sets 30–60 m at 90–100% x 5 repetitions for Start Dash and (250–300 m at 90%) 3–5 repetitions, 50–100 m at a constant tempo for Skip 3–5 repetitions	50–100 m 5 kg Weights 2 repetitions on Sled for Resistance Running 150 m at 90% 3 repetitions 2–3 sets (150–200 m at 85%) 5 repetitions, 50 m at a constant tempo for Skip x 5 repetitions 250–300 m at 90% 3 repetitions 1–2 set (200–300 m at 85%) 3–5 repetitions 50–100 m at a constant tempo for Skip 3–5 repetitions

**The sprinters practiced as a sprint training of either content during each phase.*
**Percentage represents the rate of increase in running velocity.*

Table 3.
Contents of usual sprint training for submaximal and maximal running.

followed by acute fatigue. Usual training helps sprinters achieve submaximal and maximal running speed by repeated acute fatigue, which causes an adaptive response. Submaximal running and maximal running were practiced with independent efforts (non-assisted) or under an increased workload, such as running uphill or using a sled (resisted). Therefore, the usual training for submaximal and maximal running comprises several runs (**Table 3**).

5.2.4 Supramaximal running for quality training

Supramaximal running is a type of quality training. Therefore, this training was conducted at that point in the overall sprint training schedule when the quality was improved or when it was high. Moreover, the total volume of training decreased (**Figure 5**).

Supramaximal running for special training was practiced with assistance in tow training. Tow training was performed using a towing machine (**Figure 6**) and a rubber tube [6, 25, 45]. The rate of increase in the velocity of a sprinter is up to 103–107% during supramaximal running [45–50]. In sprinters, the generated higher force with overspeed training is postulated to be related to hamstring injuries in supramaximal running. The researchers and coaches have highlighted issues related to hamstring injuries [50–52].

On the other hand, muscle fatigue is a risk factor for hamstring injuries [33, 53, 54]. Therefore, supramaximal running was performed following a day off or on an individual practice day when the lowest muscle fatigue was expected. Each sprinter was involved in 2–5 runs/day for 15–25 days/season. In reality, over a season, the number of runs per sprinter ranged from 20 to 30. Special sprint training for supramaximal running includes a few runs (**Table 4**).

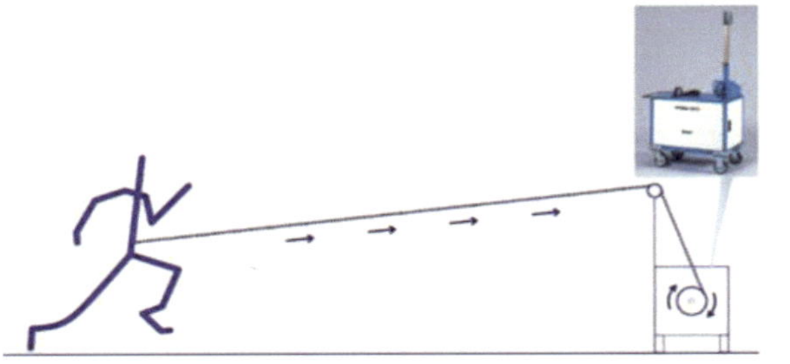

Figure 6.
Supramaximal running in towing system.

Training Contents	
Pre-season and 1 st season:⑤	**1st, 2nd and Inter-season:⑥,⑦**
50–100 m at 105% × 3–5 repetition	50 m at 105–110% × 3 repetition 50 m at 105–110% × 1

**The sprinters selected the distanse, the rate of increase in running velocity and numbers in towing during each phase.*

Table 4.
Contents of special sprint training for supramaximal running.

5.2.5 Effective strategic combination programs to prevent hamstring injuries

The injury risk increases in fatigue conditions [53, 54]. Fatigue conditions may lead to dys-synergic contraction of different muscle groups, lack of muscle strength, and decreased muscle endurance causing hamstring injuries [33]. Therefore, supramaximal runs were practiced with fewer repetitions because of the fatigued states of the sprinters. The effective strategic combination of prevention programs, agility, strength, and flexibility could reduce the incidence of hamstring injuries (**Figure** 7).

Agility program allows learning the rapid motion needed to cope with supramaximal running. Sprinters who practiced using ladders and mini-hurdles exhibited rapid stepping equivalent to or faster than the stride frequency that had been observed during supramaximal running [6]. Motion training at a high level, such as supramaximal running, which requires a quick sprinting motion, incorporates the learning of new muscle recruitment patterns that involve peripheral sensory input. The muscle synergy adapted to high-level sprinting motion was likely acquired by all sprinters using ladders and mini-hurdles. Thus, the incidence of hamstring injuries decreased during supramaximal running.

Strength program applies an eccentric load to the hamstring through the trunk position at the injury position. During supramaximal training, eccentric strength program worked well against load on the hamstrings. The incidence of hamstring injuries during period III with eccentric strength program decreased compared with the period I. All sprinters strengthened their hamstrings with leg curls, hip extensions, and two types of modified Nordic hamstring exercises. This likely decreased the incidence of hamstring injuries during supramaximal running.

With dynamic stretching, the neuromuscular system becomes a softer musculotendinous system with increased length and allows the performance of larger

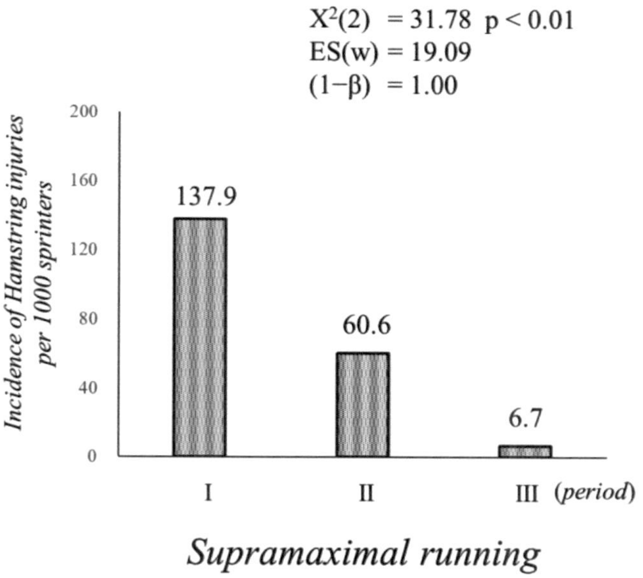

Figure 7.
Hamstring injury rate during supramaximal running.

movements [55]. The goal of dynamic stretching is to provide flexibility in the lumbopelvic region muscles. Moreover, it adapts the hip joint to a mobile state where dynamic flexibility is secured. The hip joint movement adapted to supramaximal running may be acquired by stretching the hamstring, quadriceps femoris, and other muscles during active joint movements. Dynamic stretching is conjectured to function effectively in preventing hamstring injuries while assisting athletes to perform at a high level. Dynamic stretching is potentially effective in preventing hamstring injuries in supramaximal running.

By implementing three hamstring injury programs simultaneously—agility, strength, and flexibility—we can demonstrate their relative effects on injury reduction. Therefore, investigating what program or combination is the most effective is necessary. The combination of prevention programs, agility, strength, and flexibility, reduced the incidences of hamstring injuries. The prevention program was effective in supramaximal running because only a few runs were made due to the fatigued states of the sprinter.

5.2.6 Muscle fatigue condition: a crucial risk factor for hamstring injuries

Usual training has sufficient volume and intensity to cause overload, followed by acute fatigue [19]. The yearly summation of several training programs will result in greater fatigue and subsequent supercompensation response [56]. This adaptive response will leave the participant in a healthier state than the previous state [56]. Therefore, usual sprint training for submaximal and maximal running contains several runs. Even if the program could prevent hamstring injuries during submaximal/maximal running with a sufficient volume for several runs in usual training, the incidence of hamstring injuries did not decrease (**Figure 8**).

Fatigue has an impact on muscle activation and function, including lumbopelvic control, knee stability, leg stiffness, and muscle-tendon unit energy transfer [53].

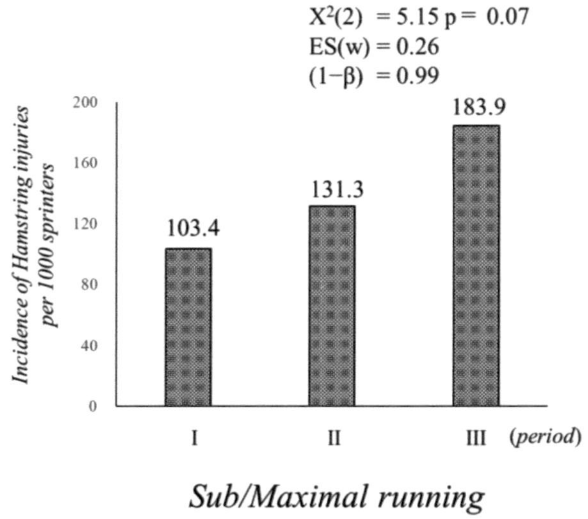

Figure 8.
Hamstring injury rate during submaximal and maximal running.

Alterations in running kinematics, such as the "Groucho position" caused by fatigue, minimize exercise efficiency while elevating force moments. Additionally, it is associated with increased stress on contractile muscle units. Theoretically, there is a risk of damage to the hamstrings [53].

In usual training, which causes muscle fatigue following several runs, the physical performance of increased strength, agility, and flexibility with prevention programs may not have positive effects on hamstring activation and function. Hamstring injury prevention program had no effect on the fatigued hamstrings, muscle groups, hip extensors, and knee flexors.

6. Practical applications

The combination of three programs, agility, strength, and flexibility contributes well to sprinters for the prevention of muscle injuries. Moreover, the prescription should consider conditioning depending on sprinters.

In running-based training, clarifying and considering the time set for a distance are important to not only improve performance but also prevent injuries. In usual training for several runs, it is difficult to clear the set time because of fatigue caused by repeated running. At that time, "Groucho running" patterns may be observed because of poor muscle activation and function [53]. A sprinter unable to clear the time set by the coach will not achieve the training purpose. Therefore, for running-based training, sprinters should carefully monitor the running time and inform the training load so that the athletes are objectively exposed to the appropriate training volume [54].

Furthermore, it is also important to subjectively consider fatigue. Coaches should check the physical condition (degree of fatigue) of the sprinters before training using a numerical value (e.g., visual analog scale) to quantify the physical condition of the sprinters (**Table 4**). Sprinters should measure body temperature, heart rate, and flexibility in the morning daily and translate their values into subjective physical condition on a scale

Subjective Scale	Physical Condition
1	Very Bad
2	Bad
3	Neither Bad or Good
4	Good
5	Very Good

Sprinters measure body temperature, heart rate, and flexibility in the morning on every day, translate their values into subjective physical condition on a scale of 1–5.
Sprinters rate themselves scale 1 or 2 when they experience the muscle pain or tightness. Then, the coach makes sprinters stop training or practice training with quality and volume adjustment.
Sprinters often rate themselves scale 3 or 4.
Sprinters rate themselves scale 5 that is led by peaking for a match.

Table 5.
Subjective scale for physical condition for sprinters.

of 1 (very bad) to 5 (very good). If sprinters rate themselves as a scale 1 or 2 when they experience muscle pain or tightness, then their coach can make sprinters stop training or practice training with quality and volume adjustment. Sprinters often rate themselves as scale 3 or 4. Sprinters rate themselves as 5 that is led by peaking for a match.

Coaches, trainers, and sports doctors encourage sprinters in training cessation for objective and subjective monitoring of the degree of fatigue and to avoid the risk of injuries.

To date, the usefulness of measuring muscle stiffness for muscle fatigue has been studied [57]. It has been reported that muscle stiffness increases by performing fatigue tasks [58]. In recent years, new technologies have made it possible to measure muscles stiffness [59]. It may be an effective means for objective assessment of the daily, weekly, and seasonal muscle condition of a sprinter (**Table 5**).

Furthermore, hamstring injury programs should include high-intensity aerobic exercises during the basic training period [60] as previous papers demonstrated the presence of strength-endurance deficits by these injuries [61]. The overall improvement in fitness levels minimizes the fatigue burden [54].

Regardless of the training efficacy, the presence of risk factors makes the program unacceptable. Therefore, monitoring is necessary to ensure the efficacy of provided training without spikes in training load or any risks for hamstring injuries [54].

7. Implications and future directions

The more sprint performance improves, the higher the incidence of hamstring injuries [16, 26], and it is still higher in elite sprinters. A hamstring prevention program is possible by building a support system for program methods (contents) with techniques and strategies based on data accumulation and cooperation of coaches, researchers, trainers, and sports doctors (**Figure 9**).

Future research should verify the effectiveness of this preventive program for hamstring injuries in sprinters. In addition, for more effective prevention, nonmodifiable factors such as anterior pelvic tilt, fiber-type distribution, and previous injury [62] may have been taken into consideration during program execution [6].

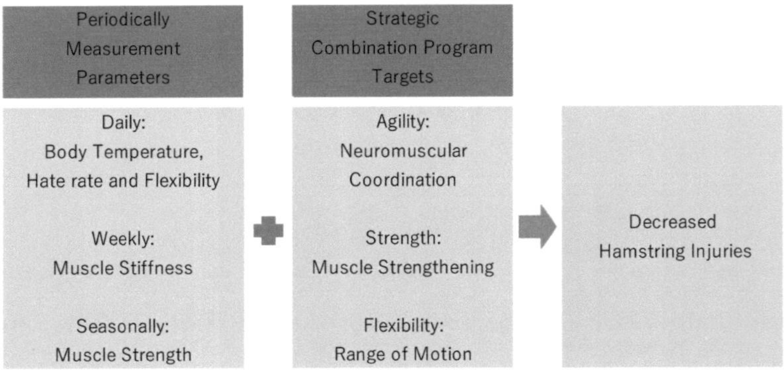

Figure 9.
Ideal hamstring injury prevention program for sprinters.

Conflict of interest

The authors declare no conflict of interest.

Author details

Yusaku Sugiura[1*], Yuji Takazawa[2], Kazuhiko Yamazaki[3] and Kazuhiko Sakuma[4]

1 Sport Science, Meikai University, Urayasu, Japan

2 Department of Sports Medicine, Graduate School of Medicine, Health and Sports Science, Juntendo University, Tokyo, Japan

3 Graduate School of Health and Sports Science, Juntendo University, Inzai, Japan

4 Former Graduate School of Health and Sports Science, Juntendo University, Inzai, Japan

*Address all correspondence to: yusaku@meikai.ac.jp

References

[1] Mero A, Komi PV. Effects of supramaximal velocity on biomechanical variables in sprinting. Journal of Applied Biomechanics. 1985;**1**:240-252. DOI: 10.1123/ijsb.1.3.240

[2] Ae M, Miyashita K, Yokoi T, Hashihara Y. Mechanical power and work done by the muscle of the lower limb during running at different speeds. Biomechanics X-B 1987, 6. J Biomech Kinetic limitations of maximal sprinting speed. 1983;**16**(79-83):895-899. DOI: 10.1016/0021-9290(83)90048-9

[3] Chapman AE, Caldwell GE. Kinetic limitations of maximal sprinting speed. Journal of Biomechanics. 1983;**16**:79-83

[4] Mann RV. A kinetic analysis of sprinting. Medicine and Science in Sports and Exercise. 1981;**13**(5):325-328. DOI: 10.1249/00005768-198105000-00010

[5] Dalton SL, Kerr ZY, Dompier TP. Epidemiology of hamstring strains in 25 NCAA sports in the 20092010 to 20132014 academic years. The American Journal of Sports Medicine. 2015;**43**(11):2671-2679. DOI: 10.1177/0363546515599631

[6] Sugiura Y, Sakuma K, Sakuraba K, Sato Y. Prevention of hamstring injuries in collegiate sprinters. Orthopaedic Journal of Sports Medicine. 2017;**5**(1):2325967116681524. DOI: 10.1177/2325967116681524

[7] Brukner P, Khan K. Clinical Sports Medicine. 3rd ed. New Zealand, Australia: McGraw-Hill Medical; 2009

[8] Van der Made AD, Wieldraaijer T, Kerkhoffs GM, Kleipool RP, Engebretsen L, van Dijk CN, et al. The hamstring muscle complex. Knee Surgery, Sports Traumatology, Arthroscopy. 2015;**23**(7):2115-2122. DOI: 10.1007/s00167-013-2744-0

[9] Woodley SJ, Storey RN. Review of hamstring anatomy. Aspetar Sports Medicine Journal. 2013;**2**:432-437

[10] Burkett LN. Investigation into hamstring strains: The case of the hybrid muscle. The Journal of Sports Medicine. 1975;**3**(5):228-231. DOI: 10.1177/036354657500300504

[11] Clanton TO, Coupe KJ. Hamstring Straing in athletes; diagnosis and treatment. The Journal of the American Academy of Orthopaedic Surgeons. 1998;**6**(4):237-248. DOI: 10.5435/00124635-199807000-00005

[12] Pollock N, Kelly S, Lee J, Stone B, Giakoumis M, Polglass G, et al. A 4-year study of hamstring injury outcomes in elite track and field using the British athletics rehabilitation approach. British Journal of Sports Medicine. 2022;**56**(5):257-263. DOI: 10.1136/bjsports-2020-103791

[13] Pollock N, James SLJ, Lee JC, Chakraverty R. British athletics muscle injury classification: A new grading system. British Journal of Sports Medicine. 2014;**48**(18):1347-1351. DOI: 10.1136/bjsports-2013-093302

[14] Simonsen EB, Thomsen L, Klausen K. Activity of mono-and biarticular leg muscles during sprint running. European Journal of Applied Physiology and Occupational Physiology. 1985;**54**(5): 524-532. DOI: 10.1007/BF00422964

[15] Stanton P. Hamstring injuries and eccentric exercise. EXCEL. 1986;**3**:13-15

[16] Stanton P, Purdham C. Hamstring injuries in sprinting—The role of eccentric exercise. The Journal of Orthopaedic and Sports Physical Therapy. 1989;**10**(9):343-349. DOI: 10.2519/jospt.1989.10.9.343

[17] Jonkers I, Stewart C, Spaepen A. The complementary role of the plantarflexors, hamstrings and gluteus maximus in the control of stance limb stability during gait. Gait & Posture. 2003;**17**(3):264-272. DOI: 10.1016/s0966-6362(02)00102-9

[18] Schache AG, Dorn TW, Blanch PD, Brown NA, Pandy MG. Mechanics of the human hamstring muscles during sprinting. Medicine and Science in Sports and Exercise. 2012;**44**(4):647-658. DOI: 10.1249/MSS.0b013e318236a3d2

[19] Sugiura Y, Sakuma K, Fujita S, Aoki K, Takazawa Y. Effects of various numbers of runs on the success of hamstring injury prevention program in sprinters. International Journal of Environmental Research and Public Health. 2022;**19**(15):9373. DOI: 10.3390/ijerph19159375

[20] Howard RM, Conway R, Harrison AJ. Muscle activity in sprinting: A review. Sports Biomechanics. 2018;**17**(1):1-17. DOI: 10.1080/14763141.2016.1252790

[21] Orchard J. Biomechanics of muscle strain injury. N Z J Sports Med. 2002;**30**:92-98

[22] Clanton TO, Coupe KJ. Hamsting strains in athletes: Diagnosis and treatment. The Journal of the American Academy of Orthopaedic Surgeons. 1998;**6**(4):237-248. DOI:10.5435/00124635-199807000-00005

[23] Alonso J, McHugh MP, Mullaney MJ, Tyler TF. Effect of hamstring flexibility on isometric knee flexion angle-torque relationship. Scandinavian Journal of Medicine & Science in Sports. 2009;**19**(2):252-256. DOI: 10.1111/j.1600-0838.2008.00792.x

[24] Mann R, Sprague P. A kinetic analysis of the ground leg during sprint running. Research Quarterly for Exercise and Sport. 1980;**51**(2):334-348. DOI: 10.1080/02701367.1980.10605202

[25] Sugiura Y, Sakuma K, Fujita S, Sakuraba K. Hamstring injury prevention program and recommendation for stride frequency during tow-training optimization. Applied Sciences. 2021;**11**(14):6500. DOI: 10.3390/app11146500

[26] Jönhagen S, Németh G, Eriksson E. Hamstring injuries in sprinters. The role of concentric and eccentric hamstring muscle strength and flexibility. The American Journal of Sports Medicine. 1994;**22**(2):262-266. DOI: 10.1177/036354659402200218

[27] Lysholm J, Wiklander J. Injuries in runners. The American Journal of Sports Medicine. 1987;**15**(2):168-171. DOI: 10.1177/036354658701500213

[28] Chumanov ES, Heiderscheit BC, Thelen DG. Hamstring musculotendon dynamics during stance and swing phases of high-speed running. Medicine and Science in Sports and Exercise. 2011;**43**(3):525-532. DOI: 10.1249/MSS.0b013e3181f23fe8

[29] Fiorentino NM, Rehorn MR, Chumanov ES, Thelen DG, Blemker SS. Computational models predict larger muscle tissue strains at faster sprinting speeds. Medicine and Science in Sports and Exercise. 2014;**46**(4):776-786. DOI: 10.1249/MSS.0000000000000172

[30] Heiderscheit BC, Hoerth DM, Chumanov ES, Swanson SC, Thelen BJ,

Thelen DG. Identifying the time of occurrence of a hamstring strain injury during treadmill running: A case study. Clinical Biomechanics (Bristol Avon). 2005;**20**(10):1072-1078. DOI: 10.1016/j.clinbiomech.2005.07.005

[31] Higashihara A, Nagano Y, Ono T, Fukubayashi T. Relationship between the peak time of hamstring stretch and activation during sprinting. European Journal of Sport Science. 2016;**16**(1):36-41. DOI: 10.1080/17461391.2014.973913

[32] Schache AG, Wrigley TV, Baker R, Pandy MG. Biomechanical response to hamstring muscle strain injury. Gait & Posture. 2009;**29**(2):332-338. DOI: 10.1016/j.gaitpost.2008.10.054

[33] Agre JC. Hamstring injuries. Proposed aetiological factors, prevention, and treatment. Sports Medicine. 1985;**2**(1):21-33. DOI: 10.2165/00007256-198502010-00003

[34] Worrell TW. Factors associated with hamstring injuries: An approach to treatment and preventative measures. Sports Medicine. 1994;**17**(5):338-345. DOI: 10.2165/00007256-199417050-00006

[35] Devlin L. Recurrent posterior thigh symptoms detrimental to performance in rugby union: Predisposing factors. Sports Medicine. 2000;**29**(4):273-287. DOI: 10.2165/00007256-200029040-00005

[36] Proske U, Morgan DL, Brockett CL, Percival P. Identifying athletes at risk of hamstring strains and how to protect them. Clinical and Experimental Pharmacology & Physiology. 2004;**31**(8):546-550. DOI: 10.1111/j.1440-1681.2004.04028.x

[37] Sugiura Y, Saito T, Sakuraba K, Sakuma K, Suzuki E. Strength deficits identified with concentric action of the hip extensors and eccentric action of the hamstrings predispose to hamstring injuryin elite sprinters. The Journal of Orthopaedic and Sports Physical Therapy. 2008;**38**(8):457-464. DOI: 10.2519/jospt.2008.2575

[38] Brockett CL, Morgan DL, Proske U. Human hamstring muscles adapt to eccentric exercise by changing optimum length. Medicine and Science in Sports and Exercise. 2001;**33**(5):783-790. DOI: 10.1097/00005768-200105000-00017

[39] Ekstrand J, Gillquist J. Soccer injuries and their mechanisms: A prospective study. Medicine and Science in Sports and Exercise. 1983;**15**(3):267-270. DOI: 10.1249/00005768-198315030-00014

[40] Askling CM, Tengvar M, Thorstensson A. Acute hamstring injuries in Swedish elite football: Aprospective randomised controlled clinical trial comparing two rehabilitation protocols. British Journal of Sports Medicine. 2013;**47**(15):953-959. DOI: 10.1136/bjsports-2013-092165

[41] Heiderscheit BC, Sherry MA, Silder A, Chumanov ES, Thelen DG. Hamstring strain injuries: Recommendations for diagnosis, rehabilitation, and injury prevention. The Journal of Orthopaedic and Sports Physical Therapy. 2010;**40**(2):67-81. DOI: 10.2519/jospt.2010.3047

[42] Arnason A, Andersen TE, Holme I, Engebretsen L, Bahr R. Prevention of hamstring strains in elite soccer: An intervention study. Scandinavian Journal of Medicine & Science in Sports. 2008;**18**(1):40-48. DOI: 10.1111/j.1600-0838.2006.00634.x

[43] Mjølsnes R, Arnason A, Østhagen T, Raastad T, Bahr RAA.

A 10-week randomized trial comparing eccentric vs. concentric hamstring strength training in well-trained soccer players. Scandinavian Journal of Medicine & Science in Sports. 2004;**14**(5):311-317. DOI: 10.1046/j.1600-0838.2003.367.x

[44] Joyce D, Lewindon D. Retraining the injured athlete. In: Joyce D, Lewindon D, editors. High-Performance Training for Sports. Champaign, IL: Human Kinetics Publishers; 2014. pp. 85-96

[45] Sugiura Y, Aoki J. Effects of supramaximal running on stride frequency and stride length in sprinters. Advances in Exercise and Sports Physiology. 2008;**14**:9-17

[46] Ae M, Itoh N, Muraki Y, Miyashita K. Optimal tension of isotonic towing for sprint training. In: Proceedings of the XV Congress of International Society of Biomechanics. Jyvaskyla, Finland; 1995

[47] Ito N. Effects of towing system used a pulley on sprinting. Sprint Res. 1998;**8**:29-37 (In Japanese)

[48] Sugiura Y, Migita T, Sakuraba K, Sakuma K, Aoki J. Effects of tow training on delayed-onset muscle soreness and serum CK activity for sprinters who are accustomed to supramaximal running. Jpn J Clin Sports Med. 2009;**17**:247-254 (In Japanese)

[49] Mero A, Komi PV. Force-, EMG-, and elasticity-velocity relationships at submaximal, maximal and supramaximal running speeds in sprinters. European Journal of Applied Physiology and Occupational Physiology. 1986;**55**(5):553-561. DOI: 10.1007/BF00421652

[50] Dintiman GB. Training the sprinter. In: Cooper JM, editor. What Research Tells the Coach about Sprinting. Reston, VA: AAHPER Publications; 1974. pp. 49-81

[51] Hicks D. Resisted and assisted sprint training: Determining the transfer to maximal sprinting. New Studies In Athletics. 2018;**32**:35-51

[52] Mero A, Komi PV, Rusko H, Hirvonen J. Neuromuscular and anaerobic performance of sprinters at maximal and supramaximal speed. International Journal of Sports Medicine. 1987;**8**(Suppl. 1):55-60. DOI: 10.1055/s-2008-1025704

[53] Huygaerts S, Cos F, Cohen DD, Calleja-González J, Guitart M, Blazevich AJ, et al. Mechanisms of hamstring strain injury: Interactions between fatigue, muscle Activationand function. Sports. 2020;**8**(5):65. DOI: 10.3390/sports8050065

[54] Wing C, Bishop C. Hamstring strain injuries: Incidence, mechanisms, risk factors, and training recommendations. Strength & Conditioning Journal. 2020;**42**(3):40-57. DOI: 10.1519/SSC.0000000000000538

[55] Papadopoulos GST, Siatras T, Kellis S. The effect of static and dynamic stretching exercises on the maximal isokinetic strength of the knee extensors and flexors. Isokinetics and Exercise Science. 2005;**13**(4):285-291. DOI: 10.3233/IES-2005-0216

[56] Rosenblett B. Planning a performance programme. In: Joyce D, Lewindon D, editors. High-Performance Training for Sports. Champaign, IL: Human Kinetics Publishers; 2014. p. 247

[57] Witte RS, Kim K, Martin BJ, O'Donnell M. Effect of fatigue on muscle elasticity in the human forearm using ultrasound strain imaging. In: Conf Proc IEEE Eng Med Biol Soc. Proceedings of

the Annu Int Conf IEEE Eng Med Biol Soc Annu Conf. Piscataway, NJ: IEEE Service Center; 2006. pp. 4490-4493. DOI: 10.1109/IEMBS.2006.260850

[58] Bouillard K, Jubeau M, Nordez A, Hug F. Effect of vastus lateral is fatigue on load sharing between quadriceps femoris muscles during isometric knee extensions. Journal of Neurophysiology. 2014;**111**(4):768-776

[59] Miyamoto N, Hirata K, Inoue K, Hashimoto T. Muscle stiffness of the vastus lateralis in sprinters and long-distance runners. Medicine and Science in Sports and Exercise. 2019;**51**(10):2080-2087. DOI: 10.1249/MSS.0000000000002024

[60] Baker D. Recent trends in high-intensity aerobic training for field sports. Proof Strength Cond. 2011;**22**:38

[61] Lord C, Ma'ayah F, AJAJ B. Change in knee flexor torque after fatiguing exercise identifies previous hamstring injury in football players. Scandinavian Journal of Medicine & Science in Sports. 2018;**28**(3):1235-1243. DOI: 10.1111/sms.13007

[62] Opar DA, Williams MD, Shield AJ. Hamstring strain injuries: Factors that lead to injury and re-injury. Sports Medicine. 2012;**42**(3):209-226. DOI: 10.2165/11594800-000000000-00000

Chapter 3

Playing Surface and Injury Risk: Artificial Turf Vs. Natural Grass

Griffith G. Gosnell, Brett A. Gerber, Gregory P. Guyton and Heath P. Gould

Abstract

Artificial turf's developmental history spans 6 generations and includes design improvements that transformed an injury-inducing 1st generation field into a modern 3rd generation natural grass substitute. Artificial turf has become a widely adopted playing surface with a $2.7 billion United States Dollar (USD) valuation in North America. Turf's popularity is due to its increased functionality and decreased cost compared to natural grass that allows more sports to play on the surface for longer time periods with decreased maintenance costs. From a biomechanical perspective, artificial turf exhibits higher frictional coefficients than natural grass resulting in higher foot and ankle injury rates. Concussion rates on turf are decreased compared to natural grass due to lower G-max values on well-maintained artificial surfaces. Hip, knee, and overall injury rates are equivalent between the two surfaces except in specific populations including elite-level American football players that exhibit increased knee injury rates on artificial turf. Due to these tradeoffs, the authors suggest that athletic organizations with funding to support professional groundskeeping should consider investing in natural grass due to athlete preference and decreased injury risk. In contrast, organizations without sufficient funding for professional groundskeeping operations may consider investing in modern artificial turf due to its associated long-term benefits and decreased costs.

Keywords: artificial turf, synthetic turf, natural grass, sport fields, playing surfaces, comparative injury rates, lower extremity injuries, concussions

1. Introduction

1.1 The problem at large

Injury reduction studies and the strategies such studies create are important methods used to protect amateur and professional athletes worldwide. Through the process of identifying risk factors and taking steps to mitigate them, researchers and athletic administrators can take active roles in athlete safety. In the United States (US) alone, 2.6 million sports-related emergency room visits occur each year for patients in the 5–25 age range. Such injury rates account for significant financial and time costs for athletes and medical personnel, as US high-school athletics result in 500,000 medical visits, 30,000 hospitalizations, and $2 billion USD costs to the US healthcare system on average per year [1]. A study of North Carolina high school athletes demonstrated that injury-related expenses including medical costs, lost opportunity costs, and estimated impact on quality of life totaled an average of $10,432 USD per injury [2]. Due to the substantial impact of these athletic injuries at a personal and societal level, debates continue to occur regarding the specific equipment, protocols, and playing surfaces that will maximize player safety and minimize risk of injury. In this chapter, we compare athletic injury rates between artificial turf and natural grass playing surfaces. We set out to provide a concise summary and synthesis of the available literature, in hopes that this information may be useful to both medical providers and athletic administrators who are involved in the care of athletes across all levels of play.

1.2 History of artificial turf

The 1st artificial turf field was installed in 1966 in the Houston Astrodome in Houston, Texas [3]. Produced by Monsanto and named AstroTurf, this turf generation's design consisted of a thin nylon fiber woven carpet installed over top a compacted soil base [3, 4]. In 1969, 3 M produced its own but similar product, Tartan Turf, as a direct competitor to Astroturf which was subsequently installed that summer in the University of Michigan football stadium [4]. Both Astroturf and Tartan Turf are considered 1st generation turf fields due to their design and material commonalities. This 1st generation design was associated with common skin abrasions, ankle sprains due to the prevalent intersectional seams and high friction level of the woven carpet, and other injuries due to the non-forgiving solidity of the base material [3–9]. Because of these problems, the 2nd generation of artificial turf, Shag Turf, quickly evolved and came into use by 1976 [10, 11]. 2nd generation turf improved upon the prior design by adding a shock-absorbing rubber pad over the compacted soil and replacing the original carpet with vertically positioned polypropylene fibers supported in a silica-sand infill [3–7]. This design aided the athletic experience through providing a flatter and more routine playing surface that mimicked natural grass fields to a higher degree. Unfortunately, these fields exhibited a high propensity to cause serious abrasions to players, which significantly limited their adoption among American football and soccer organizations [3, 5, 7, 10–12]. This led to the genesis of 3rd generation artificial turf. First installed in a Pennsylvania high school in 1997, the design took cues from the 2nd generation but with a greater focus on athlete safety [3, 13]. Changes between the 2nd and 3rd generation included altering the fiber composition from polypropylene to polyethylene to decrease skin abrasions, increasing fiber length, and spreading the fibers laterally to rely more heavily on the infill material for structural support and to decrease surface hardness [3, 5, 14]. The infill material was made into a deeper layer and switched from silica sand to crumb rubber or a mixture of both elements, occasionally also combined with other infill materials such as different elastomers, polymers, and organic materials such as coconut fibers, cork, and ground walnut shells [3]. These changes were made to increase the shock absorbing properties of the playing surface to increase player safety and improve agility as well as ball handling characteristics. Technically, additional generations of turf exist but their validity remains debated. Companies have claimed development of 4th, 5th, and 6th generation artificial turf which all essentially build on the same principles of 3rd generation turf, but use specific materials or manufacturing processes that eliminate the need for rubber infill. These claims remain debated due to the notion that 4th, 5th, and 6th generation turf exist only as marketing ploys used by companies to promote their products as novel developments, when in reality their design borrows heavily from 3rd generation turf characteristics [15–17]. Currently, the authors are not aware of any major athletic regulatory bodies that recognize these designs as unique turf generations, making 3rd generation artificial turf the current industry standard for modern turf design.

Today, artificial turf's success is represented in its wide adoption at all levels and types of athletic competition. In North America alone in 2020, the total value of synthetic turf fields was estimated at $2.7 billion USD with a total area of 265 million square feet and 436 million pounds of infill material installed [18]. Out of 32 National Football League teams, 16 use turf fields across 14 stadiums [19]. With this high degree of use, comparison of injury risks between artificial turf and natural grass fields could provide applicable information that has the potential to effect millions of athletes every year.

1.3 Cost of artificial turf vs. grass injuries

Artificial turf is generally installed as a cost-saving, functional enhancement to athletic facilities for its ability to host multiple sports on the same field with minimal repair time and lower maintenance costs in comparison to natural grass fields. A common misconception surrounding artificial turf is its zero-maintenance nature. While artificial turf certainly has a lower maintenance cost than natural grass, it still requires a substantial level of upkeep to maintain the surface. Examples of such maintenance include debris removal, sanitation and disinfection, watering for heat dispersion, field hardness testing and infill replacement, rake sweeping and dragging to maintain proper fiber alignment and G-max value, snow removal in the winter, and regular certification checks to ensure maintenance is keeping the field within specification parameters [20, 21]. Even with these maintenance requirements and their associated costs, artificial turf still remains a significantly more cost effective option in the long term.

An analysis conducted by a field turf industry representative comparing the cost differential for an artificial versus natural grass 80,000 square foot field notes this cost disparity. Whereas artificial turf has considerably higher initial installation costs of $320,000 for base preparation and $400,000 for materials, maintenance costs of only $5000 per year significantly drop the long-term price compared to that of a natural grass field with costs of $150,000 for base preparation; $200,000 for materials; and $20,000 annual maintenance costs [6, 22]. Factoring in the significant increase in useable hours afforded by an artificial turf field, the 10-year average cost per hour of use for a turf field is estimated to be $25.74 whereas that of a natural grass field is over 3 times higher at $91.20 [6, 22]. Although these figures were sourced from turf industry representatives with potential for bias to promote the widespread adoption of turf, these analyses provide a general idea of possible financial savings associated with artificial playing surfaces.

1.4 Biomechanical factors

To understand and investigate the injuries associated with playing surface type, we must also understand the biomechanical factors at play that have a role in causing such injuries. At a base level, these factors can be split into two groups - intrinsic factors and extrinsic factors. Intrinsic factors pertain to the athlete and include body weight, velocity, acceleration, deceleration, angle of the athlete's foot and height before contact. Extrinsic factors pertain to variables outside of the athlete including cleat or shoe design, type of playing surface, and environmental aspects [6, 8]. Physics principles also play a role in athlete risk and safety through concepts such as coefficient of friction (COF), coefficient of release, coefficient of restitution and associated G-max value, and rotational stiffness (**Table 1**) [6, 8, 14, 24]. These principles and their impact on the athlete exist, for the most part, in the interaction between the playing surface and the athlete's footwear.

Athlete shoe or cleat choice plays a critical role in determining the biomechanical characteristics involved between the playing surface and their feet. As a general rule, cleats of any type exhibit higher COF, coefficient of release, and peak torque than their shoe counterparts when on an artificial turf surface [6, 27–31]. This concept is also applicable on grass surfaces, although the COF, coefficient of release, and peak torque values are decreased for each respective shoe type [28, 32, 33]. Comparatively, turf shoes, specifically designed to only be worn on old generation carpet-like turf, exhibit the highest COF and coefficient of release of any shoe-surface combination [34]. Longer length and larger diameter spikes on cleat bottoms also produce higher friction rates, torque rates, and rotational stiffness than cleats with shorter or narrower spikes [23]. Friction and torque are also further influenced by cleat layout. Cleat layouts with a higher concentration of spikes on forefoot exhibit higher torques on average compared to designs with more spikes on the hindfoot [35]. Aside from the cleat layout, cleat sole stiffness may also play an important role in athlete safety and performance. This role is currently poorly understood, as different studies have demonstrated both beneficial and adverse effects related to cleat sole stiffness with regard to injury risk [33, 36, 37]. These contradicting results are likely due to specific characteristics pertaining to specific athletes, sports, and playing surfaces [38].

Exogenous factors such as athlete weight, weather, and surface type may further alter the foot-playing surface relationship. A prior study has demonstrated that compressive load correlates with COF, coefficient of release, and rotational stiffness regardless of shoe type [39]. This result points to greater torques being generated by larger athletes that produce higher compressive loads and could have significance in injury rates pertaining to a particular sport with larger average athlete body size [34, 39]. Field conditions and surface type further complicate this relationship, as wet and slippery fields exhibit lower frictional coefficients compared to the same fields in a dry state. Similarly, artificial turf fields are typically associated with a higher COF than grass fields, although this may be dependent on field manufacturer and field maintenance practices [40, 41]. Furthermore, objects or debris such as twigs, cleat wraps, mud, or snow obscuring the cleat spikes and thus interrupting the cleat-surface interaction can drastically decrease frictional forces [27].

As a whole, the shoe-surface interface represents a highly dynamic relationship that involves multiple factors including the athlete, shoe, and surface itself, which aggregate to establish the frictional and torque forces incurred by the athlete at each moment of competition. Field designers choosing field materials and athletes choosing cleat designs must weigh the impact of their choices between their athletic performance and risk of injury. Increased shoe-surface friction is positively related to enhanced player performance but also increases the likelihood of injury due to an athlete's foot sticking to the surface and increasing probability of twisting knee or ankle injury [34, 42, 43].

Value	Definition
Coefficient of Friction (COF)	The linear relationship of force required to slide one surface across another. Relates to how much force is required for a planted foot to slip [6, 14]
Coefficient of Release (r)	$r = \frac{Force}{Weight}$ The constant relationship, relating to static friction, that describes the peak torque applied to the shoe-surface interface. Higher values associated with higher rates of injury [6, 23]
Coefficient of Restitution	The ability for a playing surface to absorb shock. This value represents the ratio of maximum deceleration experienced by the athlete during surface impact to the normal rate of gravitational acceleration [6, 24]. This value is especially pertinent to a field's concussion risk.
G-max Value	Represents the shock-absorbing characteristics of a playing surface. As G-max increases the shock absorbing performance of the playing surface decreases. In turf fields specifically, this value increases commensurate with the field's age [25]. Playing surfaces considered safe are limited to a maximum G-max of 200 g [6, 14, 24, 26]
Rotational Stiffness	The rate at which torque develops under rotation in the shoe-playing surface interface [6]

Table 1.
Playing surface biomechanical factors.

2. Injury risk of artificial turf vs. grass playing surfaces

2.1 Overall injury risk

To determine respective injury risk of artificial turf versus natural grass fields, we refer to the systematic review conducted by Gould et al. which investigated the matter. In this review, 53 total studies were included, 24 (45.3%) studied professional athletes with the remaining 29 (54.72%) studying amateurs. 27 (50.94%) examined both practices and games while 25 (47.2%) examined only games, and 1 (1.89%) examined only practices. 29 studies (54.72%) reported on new generation artificial turf, 14 (26.42%) on old-generation turf, and 10 (18.87%) studies did not specify turf generation [44].

Overall injury rate was evaluated in 32 of these studies with 17 (53.13%) finding no difference in injury rate between the playing surfaces, 12 (37.5%) finding a higher rate on artificial turf, and 3 (9.38%) finding a higher injury rate on natural grass though all 3 of these studies were funded by representatives of artificial turf manufacturers [44]. This data is summarized below in **Figure 1**.

Artificial turf generation is an important component in determining overall injury risk. Of the studies that disclosed the turf generation, 8 studies specifically compared early generation artificial turf to natural grass and 6 (75.00%) of these studies found early generation turf to produce higher overall injury rates than their grass counterparts. Comparatively, 18 studies compared new generation artificial turf to natural grass and 13 (72.22%) found no difference in injury rates between the playing surfaces [44]. This discrepancy in study results provides evidence of the safety improvements made by each artificial turf generation, as discussed previously.

The data as a whole suggest that rates of overall injury are similar when comparing natural grass to new generation artificial turf. However new generation turf is associated with higher rates of specific injuries for specific athlete populations, which will be discussed further in subsequent sections. Early generation artificial turf is associated with higher overall injury rates for most athletes, but these playing surfaces are now largely obsolete in North America.

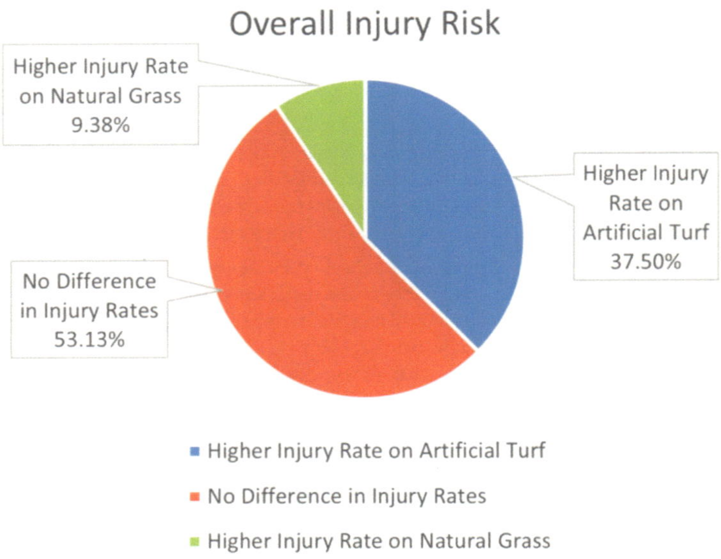

Figure 1.
Comparison of overall injury risk on artificial turf vs. natural grass.

2.2 Hip injury risk

Hip injury rate was evaluated in 13 studies with 11 (84.62%) finding no difference in hip injury rate between playing surfaces, 2 (15.38%) finding higher rates of injury on natural grass, and 0 studies finding higher rates of injury on artificial turf [44]. These results are summarized in **Figure 2** below. No studies examined injury rates on old generation artificial turf [44].

These results follow the trend of the overall injury rate in that the majority of studies find equivalent injury rates, in this case specifically pertaining to the hip, between modern 3rd generation artificial turf and natural grass fields.

2.3 Knee injury risk

Knee injury rate was evaluated in 32 studies with 19 (59.38%) finding no difference in injury rates between playing surface, 8 (25.00%) finding higher rates of injury on artificial turf, and 5 (15.63%) finding higher rates of knee injury on grass fields [44]. This data is summarized in **Figure 3**. Compared by artificial turf generation, 14/19 (73.68%) studies analyzing new generation turf found no difference in injury rates compared to grass while 4/7 (57.14%) studies analyzing old generation turf found an increased rate of knee injury on artificial surfaces [44].

Differences arose when comparing different sports to knee injury rates on each respective playing surface. Among studies involving soccer athletes, 14/16 (87.50%) found no difference between the playing surfaces. Comparatively, 8/14 (57.14%) studies examining American football found a higher rate of knee injury on artificial fields compared to grass [44]. Interestingly, 3 of the studies examining American football

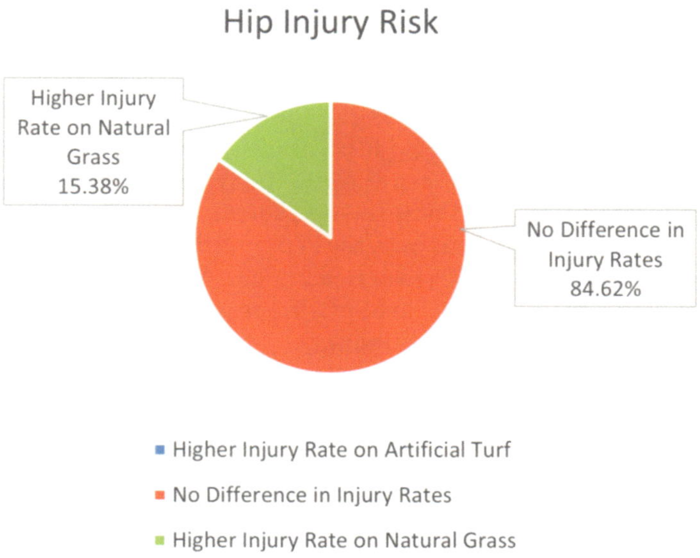

Figure 2.
Comparison of hip injury risk on artificial turf vs. natural grass.

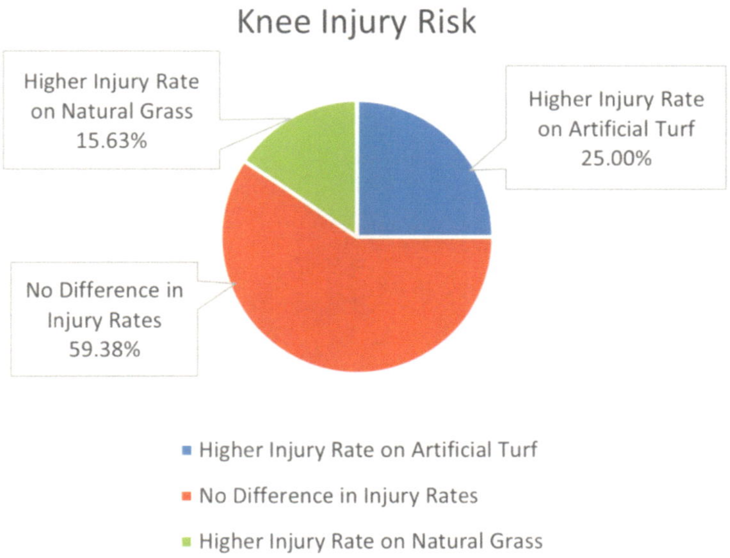

Figure 3.
Comparison of knee injury risk on artificial turf vs. natural grass.

involved new generation turf and still found a higher injury rate on the artificial surface compared to grass and all examined collegiate or professional American football players. This result stands in direct contrast to analyses covered in prior sections that showed no increased injury risk with modern turf designs. This finding may point to unknown factors that predispose elite American football players to higher knee injury risks on modern artificial turf surfaces that are not seen with other athlete types.

A possible explanation for American football players' elevated risk of knee injury follows the relationship between athlete size, applied force, and frictional coefficients. Elite American football players are typically large athletes with the average NFL cornerback weighing 193 pounds and linemen weighing 315 pounds or more [45]. Elite soccer players, in comparison, are notably smaller in stature. Measured at the 2018 FIFA World Cup, the lightest player in attendance weighed 130 pounds, the heaviest player weighed 218 pounds, and the average of the 736 players in attendance was 170 pounds [46]. This discrepancy in average athlete size may correlate to the differences in observed injury rates when viewed from a biomechanical perspective [39]. Frictional coefficients and peak torque correlate positively to applied force and thus increase in proportion to athlete size [39]. Larger football players would likely experience higher COF and torque than their smaller soccer counterparts, which could predispose them to knee injuries and therefore contribute to our described findings.

2.4 Foot and ankle injury risk

Foot and Ankle injury risk was evaluated in 25 total studies with 12 (48.00%) finding higher injury rates on artificial turf, 10 (40.00%) finding no difference in injury rates, and 3 (12.00%) finding higher injury rates on natural grass [44].

19 studies examined new-generation turf while 4 examined old generation turf. Of these studies, 9/19 (47.37%) new generation turf studies and 3/4 (75.00%) old generation turf studies found higher rates of foot and ankle injury on artificial turf compared to natural grass. This suggests that foot and ankle injury risk for all athletes on artificial turf is at least equivalent to and likely higher than rates on natural grass fields. This result is likely caused by higher COF and torque generation associated with artificial turf and is consistent with prior reviews of the topic (**Figure 4**) [44, 47–49].

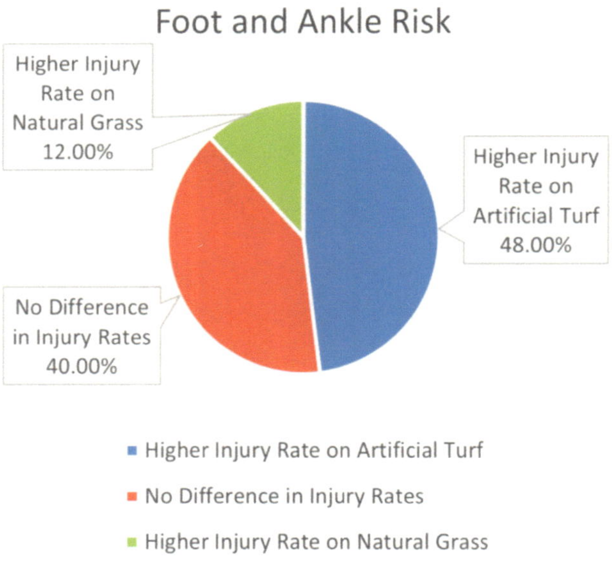

Figure 4.
Comparison of foot and ankle injury risk on artificial turf vs. natural grass.

2.5 Concussion and head injury risk

Sports-related concussion has recently become a relevant and popular research topic, with over 990 studies published in 2021 alone. Major American professional sports organizations have been at the forefront of concussion research funding and protocols, as the National Football League pledged 100 million dollars to research in 2016, and U.S. Soccer is actively testing concussion rule changes through August 2022 [50, 51]. Although there is no universal pathophysiologic definition for a concussion, it is caused by traumatic force to the head and results in immediate symptoms [52]. Therefore, variation in playing surface between artificial turf and natural grass is a logical factor to consider when determining concussion risk, particularly among contact sports where collision with playing surface may occur frequently.

A recent systematic review examined the rate ratio (RR)—ratio of the rate of injury per 1000 match playing hours on artificial turf divided by the rate of injury per 1000 match playing hours on natural grass—in soccer, American football, and rugby (**Table 2**) [53]. A rate ratio less than 1 indicates that there is a lower risk of concussion or head injury on artificial turf, whereas a rate ratio greater than 1 indicates that there is a greater risk of concussion or head injury on artificial turf. After examination of 69 observational studies to determine if they met inclusion criteria, there were a total of 12 studies published between 2004 and 2018 analyzed. Additional meta-analysis considered the subgroups of gender (male or female) and type of contact sport (soccer, American football, or rugby).

When data from all competitive contact sports is considered together, there is a lower rate of concussion or head injury on artificial turf compared to natural grass (RR = 0.89, 95% CI 0.77–1.04) [53]. In the eight studies that considered concussion only, the decreased rate of concussion on artificial turf was even more drastic (RR = 0.72, 95% CI 0.58–0.89) [53]. Together, these findings suggest that competitive contact sports on artificial turf are correlated with a reduced rate of concussion or head injury. However, it is important to consider differences in gender and sport type. For example, there was no difference in the rate of concussion or head injury on artificial turf compared to natural grass among female athletes (RR = 1.09, 95% CI 0.80–1.48) [53]. Moreover, both American football and rugby demonstrated a decreased risk of head injury or concussion on artificial turf compared to natural grass (RR = 0.72, 95% CI 0.54–0.96 and RR = 0.56, 95% CI 0.35–0.88 respectively), but soccer showed no statistical difference in rate of concussion or head injury between turf and grass (RR = 1.06, 95% CI 0.88–1.27) [53]. Whereas American football, rugby, and soccer are all considered contact sports, these data suggest that there may be more nuance in distinguishing head injury risk between contact sports. Grouping together soccer with American football and rugby for study may be problematic, as both American football and rugby regularly include violent collisions as part of the game. Although variation in the type of artificial turf should also be considered, a recent study analyzed injuries in 658 high school varsity football games and found no difference in concussion rate between artificial turf with a pad underlayer versus turf types without a pad underlayer [54].

The association of artificial turf with a reduced risk of concussion is still debated in the literature. In a survey of certified athletic trainers representing 17,459 high school and college football players, there was a disproportionately high rate of concussion and an increased risk of severe concussion among players on artificial turf compared to natural grass [55]. While less than 10% of athlete exposures were on artificial turf, almost 18% of concussions occurred on turf [55]. Moreover, 22% of head contacts on turf resulted in grade II concussions, compared to only 9% on grass, suggesting that turf-related concussions may be more severe than those occurring on grass [55]. An increased potential for

Total Number of Studies (concussion and head injury)	12
Total Number of Studies (concussion only)	8
Types of Sports	Soccer (8), American Football (2), Rugby (2)
Time Range	2004–2018
Overall Rate Ratio (concussion and head injury)	0.89, 95% CI 0.77–1.04
Overall Rate Ratio (concussion only)	0.72, 95% CI 0.58–0.89

Table 2.
Comparison of concussion and head injury risk on artificial turf vs. natural grass.

concussion on turf is supported by biomechanical factors as well, as some studies have identified higher rates of accelerometer deceleration and reduced impact attenuation on artificial turf (2558 m/s^2) compared to natural grass surfaces (2411 m/s^2) [56]. However, it is important to consider that these results are limited by the publication date of the study, as there have been significant advances in the technology of artificial turf in the last 22 years. This may influence the results toward a higher concussion rate on turf.

It is important to note that these conclusions regarding concussion and head injury are also limited by several other variables. In some sports and competitive environments, there have been substantial changes to the culture of head injury-reporting between 2000 and 2018. The type, maintenance, and temperature of both artificial turf and natural grass were also not accounted for in these study designs. Additionally, there were no studies considering American football at the professional level, so these results may not be applicable to the highest-level athletes. Finally, reported concussions may not be a result of playing surface type, as contact with the ball or other players may also result in head injury. Altogether, the most recent data suggest a greater risk of concussion on natural grass than artificial turf, but further research is warranted to draw a definitive conclusion on this topic.

3. Injury prevention strategies

3.1 Athlete-focused injury prevenion

Injury prevention is a multifactorial issue, as decreasing one category of injury risk can increase risk in other categories. This is seen with the injuries pertaining mostly to musculoskeletal categories versus surface contact injuries such as skin abrasions. Musculoskeletal injuries typically occur due to excess torque causing a locking effect on the foot [29–31, 42]. Surface contact injuries relate more to the opposite scenario in which too little grip on the field results in slipping and sliding on the surface. In this way, increasing or decreasing field friction in an attempt to decrease the rate of one type of injury may increase the incidence of a different type of injury.

Due to this scenario, a tradeoff must be considered. Athlete-focused strategies employed to decrease the rate of musculoskeletal injuries may include using cleat designs that minimize the torque placed on the lower extremities, such as cleats with spikes equally weighted in the forefoot and hindfoot or spike designs that decrease peak torque generation [30, 35]. Strategies to decrease surface contact injuries could include avoiding the use of cleat covers or any material that disrupts the shoe-surface interaction, as this can increase the risk of slipping during running and cutting movements [27, 42].

3.2 Playing surface-focused injury prevention

Injury prevention strategies focused on field design and maintenance must consider the same trade-offs described above. In general, field maintenance should be a primary focus to keep the playing surface as consistent as possible, so that athletes interact with the same surface characteristics every time. This consistency promotes both athletic performance and safety, as athletes can focus more on their sport and less on the field itself. This effect is magnified if field maintenance is lacking, as athletes are forced to play on foreign surfaces with unknown friction coefficients or, even worse, fields with different friction rates in different areas due to irregular maintenance practices.

To target specific injury rates, the strategies are similar to those discussed previously regarding augmenting specific physics principles. As a general rule, increasing field frictional coefficients will decrease field surface contact injury risk due to increased grip. However, joint injury risk may be increased in this scenario due to foot and lower limb trapping on the turf surface [27, 35, 42].

A unique factor in playing surface-focused injury prevention is the ability to protect against head and concussion injury risk. This is again accomplished with regular field maintenance, but with a focus on maintaining proper G-max values related to a field's coefficient of restitution [6, 14, 25, 26]. A safe value is typically considered below 200 G and acts as an effective way to increase athlete safety, without requiring the athlete to utilize additional equipment such as a helmet or head padding [24].

Weather changes also play a role in artificial surface properties and injury prevention, although their input is more difficult to control or mitigate. These changes may include extreme heat or cold as well as changing surface conditions with varying degrees of moisture. Depending on air conditions, artificial turf surface temperatures can be over 35 degrees Fahrenheit higher than those of a comparable natural grass field [57, 58]. Without proper preparation, such temperatures can result in diminished athletic performance and the potential for heat-related illness such as heat stroke or heat exhaustion [59]. In freezing conditions, the compacted soil sublayer in artificial turf can freeze resulting in a significantly harder surface which can increase surface contact injuries and concussions [60]. As discussed previously, environmental moisture also effects surface conditions through decreasing frictional coefficients and thus altering the foot-surface interface [27]. Some options to mitigate these concerns include indoor stadiums to maintain climate control or heated subsurface coils to minimize freeze effects [20, 61, 62].

3.3 Exercise strategies for injury prevention

Evidence-based exercise strategies allow physicians, athletic trainers, and other medical personnel to directly augment athletes' physical preparation in order to reduce the risk of injury. The FIFA 11+ Injury Prevention Program is an example of such a system that allows for medical personnel to advocate on behalf of their athletes [63, 64]. FIFA 11+ consists of a workout and warmup routine for athletes to complete several times a week, with the intention of better preparing their bodies for athletic competition and decreasing injuries. In trials, implementation of the routine was associated with a 30% reduction in non-contact injury rates among soccer athletes [63]. Such a program vetted by medical staff and supported by quantitative analysis provides a robust tool for team physicians to protect against common sports-associated injuries in a relatively straightforward and inexpensive manner. In the authors' opinion, the successful implementation of these types of programs should be a primary focus in the future. Whereas proven programs such as FIFA 11+ exist and are readily available, successfully convincing athletes to use them properly continues to be an issue. Studies of large athlete populations have found that as much as 89.3% of such populations use stretching for recovery but only 49.9% utilize such practices for pre-exercise routines, which account for the largest impact in injury prevention [65]. Maximizing the utilization of pre-exercise stretching and warmup routines would be expected to decrease the incidence of sports-related injuries and promote athlete safety moving forward.

4. Sources of bias

The validity of cost-effectiveness data and some injury studies have been impacted by industry bias and funding of private research. This presents in the form of industry-generated cost figures, which may be considered accurate in general, although the cost/benefit ratio between artificial turf and grass may be inflated to push consumers toward artificial playing surfaces. Similarly, 3 of the injury risk studies discussed in this chapter received direct funding from the artificial turf industry, and these studies consistently contradicted the majority of existing data, which does suggest some degree of study design bias in relation to funding sources. These potential biases manifested in the overall injury risk comparison, hip injury risk comparison, and foot and ankle injury risk comparison between artificial turf and natural grass [44]. Industry representatives have a vested interest in such studies, due to the financial opportunities afforded with positive research results in favor of artificial turf. A conscious effort should be made to remain aware of these studies and interpret the results in the context of these potential sources of bias.

5. Future research directions

Further research should be conducted on the biomechanical differences between modern generation turf and natural grass. Many studies included in this chapter compared early generations of artificial turf to natural grass. These investigations, if conducted again using solely modern artificial turf that mimics natural grass characteristics to a greater degree, may have found different results and more similarities between the two surfaces. Cleat design pertaining to sole stiffness should also be evaluated. At present, data in this area of study is ambiguous due to conflicting reports and should be further investigated to find the relationship between cleat stiffness, athletic performance, and injury risk [36, 37]. In addition, further studies are needed to address the gaps of understanding related to specific factors and how they interact with injury rates. Such studies may include the investigation of other sports such as field hockey and lacrosse, body mass, the use of headgear and helmets, level of athletic competition, and upper extremity injury rates. At present, comparative data in these areas are lacking and would certainly benefit from future study.

6. Conclusion

The comparison of artificial turf and natural grass suggests that injury rates are equivalent in most cases. Notable exceptions include higher rates of foot and ankle injuries in general, as well as higher knee injury rates among elite-level American football athletes, on artificial playing surfaces [44]. In contrast, concussion rates were found to be lower on artificial turf compared to natural grass. These data provide a strong indication of the importance of artificial field maintenance (specifically pertaining to G-max values) to maximize player protection and minimize the risk of field-related head injury [3, 6, 14, 20, 26]. Financial considerations suggest that artificial turf is an outstanding option for many athletic organizations, due to its low maintenance costs and higher degree of usability. Artificial fields may host a wide variety of sports that can share a single field, with a greater number of hours of use per year compared to natural grass fields [6, 22]. These factors must be weighed against the potential benefits of grass including lower musculoskeletal injury rates and an overwhelming athlete preference for a well-maintained natural grass surface, with surveys conducted by the National Football League Players Association (NFLPA) demonstrating that 69–72% of professional football players prefer natural grass to artificial turf [66–68]. Overall, the authors suggest that the use of artificial turf should be considered in organizations without adequate funding to support consistent, year-round professional grass groundskeeping. Alternatively, the authors advocate for the use of natural grass in well-funded athletic organizations (e.g. collegiate, professional), which possess appropriate funding to support professional maintenance protocols.

Conflict of interest

The authors declare no conflict of interest.

Author details

Griffith G. Gosnell[1], Brett A. Gerber[2], Gregory P. Guyton[3] and Heath P. Gould[3]*

1 Georgetown University School of Medicine, Georgetown, Washington D.C., USA

2 New York University Grossman School of Medicine, New York, USA

3 MedStar Union Memorial Hospital, Baltimore, Maryland, USA

*Address all correspondence to: heath.gould@gmail.com

References

[1] Goldberg AS, Moroz L, Smith A, Ganley T. Injury surveillance in young athletes: A clinician's guide to sports injury literature. Sports Medicine. 2007;**37**(3):265-278

[2] Knowles SB, Marshall SW, Miller T, Spicer R, Bowling JM, Loomis D, et al. Cost of injuries from a prospective cohort study of North Carolina high school athletes. Injury prevention: Journal of the International Society for Child and Adolescent Injury Prevention. 2007;**13**(6):416-421

[3] Jastifer JR, McNitt AS, Mack CD, Kent RW, McCullough KA, Coughlin MJ, et al. Synthetic turf: History, design, maintenance, and athlete safety. Sports Health. 2019;**11**(1):84-90

[4] Layden T. Artificial Turf: Change from the Ground Up. 2014. Available at: https://www.si.com/nfl/2014/05/21/nfl-history-95-objects-artificial-turf. [Accessed: July 10, 2022]

[5] Synthetic Turf History | Learn about Artificial Grass | INSTALL-IT-DIRECT. Available at: https://www.installitdirect.com/history/. [Accessed: July 7, 2022]

[6] Drakos MC, Taylor SA, Fabricant PD, Haleem AM. Synthetic playing surfaces and athlete health. The Journal of the American Academy of Orthopaedic Surgeons. 2013;**21**(5):293-302

[7] History of Artificial Sports Turf. 2021. Available at: https://www.installartificial.com/how/history-of-sports-turf. [Accessed: June 28, 2022]

[8] Fleming P. Artificial turf systems for sport surfaces: Current knowledge and research needs. Proceedings of the Institution of Mechanical Engineers, Part P: Journal of Sports Engineering and Technology. 2011;**225**(2):43-63

[9] Ekstrand J, Nigg BM. Surface-related injuries in soccer. Sports Medicine. 1989;**8**(1):56-62

[10] Albright T. Evolution of Artificial Turf. 2019. Available at: https://turfix.com/evolution-of-artificial-turf/#:~:text=In%20the%201970's%2C%20the%20second,to%20mimic%20a%20real%20grass

[11] A Brief History of Synthetic Turf. 2013. Available at: https://syntheticgrasswarehouse.com/a-brief-history-of-synthetic-turf/. [Accessed: June 29, 2022]

[12] Powell JW, Schootman M. A multivariate risk analysis of selected playing surfaces in the National Football League: 1980 to 1989. An epidemiologic study of knee injuries. The American Journal of Sports Medicine. 1992;**20**(6):686-694

[13] Stier JC, Horgan BP, Bonos SA, editors. Turfgrass: Biology, Use, and Management. Madison, WI: American Society of Agronomy: 2013 [Place of publication not identified] : Soil Science Society of America: Crop Science Society of America, 2013; 2013

[14] Drakos M. Does Artificial Turf Increase the Risk of Sports Injuries? 2008. Available at: https://www.hss.edu/conditions_artificial-turf-sports-injury-prevention.asp. [Accessed: July 7, 2022]

[15] A Guide to all Astroturf Pitches: 2G, 3G, 4G and beyond. 2019. Available at: https://www.sispitches.com/the-definitive-guide-to-all-types-of-astroturf-pitches-2g-3g-4g-and-beyond/. [Accessed: June 28, 2022]

[16] 2G, 3G, and 4G pitches. Know your playing surfaces | Playfinder Blog. 2016. Available at: https://www.playfinder.com/blog/2g-3g-4g-know-playing-surface. [Accessed: June 28, 2022]

[17] Astroturf 3rd, 4th, 5th, 6th Generation All Weather Pitches. 2012. Available at: https://www.sportsandsafetysurfaces.co.uk/blog/astroturf-3rd-4th-5th-6th-generation-all-weather-pitches/. [Accessed: June 28, 2022]

[18] About Synthetic Turf. Available at: https://www.syntheticturfcouncil.org/page/synthetic_turf. [Accessed: June 15, 2022]

[19] Which NFL Stadiums have Artificial Turf vs. Real Grass? Available at: https://www.nbcsports.com/washington/football-team/which-nfl-stadiums-have-artificial-turf-vs-real-grass. [Accessed: April 28, 2022]

[20] Jastifer JR, McNitt AS, Mack CD, Kent RW, McCullough KA, Coughlin MJ, et al. The development of mandatory practices for the testing and maintenance of synthetic turf fields in the National Football League. Int Turfgrass Soc Res J. 2021;**14**:352-363

[21] Maintenance: Synthetic Turf. Available at: https://www.safehealthyplayingfields.org/maintenance-synthetic-turf. [Accessed: April 28, 2022]

[22] Cost Analysis - Artificial Turf, Build Price - FieldTurf. Available at: https://fieldturf.com/en/why-fieldturf/cost-analysis/. [Accessed: June 14, 2022]

[23] Torg JS, Quedenfeld TC, Landau S. The shoe-surface interface and its relationship to football knee injuries. Journal of sports medicine. 1974;**2**(5):261-269

[24] ASTM International. Standard Specification for Impact Attenuation of Surfacing Materials within the Use Zone of Playground Equipment (ASTM F1292-18e1). 2020. Available at: https://www.astm.org/f1292-18e01.html

[25] g-max Testing - An Overview. Available at: http://www.turftest.com/gmax-overview.html. [Accessed: June 15, 2022]

[26] Olson H, Kennedy E. Final report for CPSC on the National Study of public playground equipment and surfacing. The National Program for Playground Safety. Report from the United States Consumer Product Safety Commission; 2018. pp. 1-18

[27] Heidt RS, Dormer SG, Cawley PW, Scranton PE, Losse G, Howard M. Differences in friction and torsional resistance in athletic shoe-turf surface interfaces. The American Journal of Sports Medicine. 1996;**24**(6):834-842

[28] Griffin LY, Agel J, Albohm MJ, Arendt EA, Dick RW, Garrett WE, et al. Noncontact anterior cruciate ligament injuries: Risk factors and prevention strategies. JAAOS - Journal of the American Academy of Orthopaedic Surgeons. 2000;**8**(3):141-150

[29] Wannop JW, Worobets JT, Stefanyshyn DJ. Footwear traction and lower extremity joint loading. The American Journal of Sports Medicine. 2010;**38**(6):1221-1228

[30] Kent R, Forman JL, Lessley D, Crandall J. The mechanics of American football cleats on natural grass and infill-type artificial playing surfaces with loads relevant to elite athletes. Sports Biomechanics. 2015;**14**(2):246-257

[31] Mack CD, Hershman EB, Anderson RB, Coughlin MJ, McNitt AS,

Sendor RR, et al. Higher rates of lower extremity injury on synthetic turf compared with natural turf among National Football League Athletes: Epidemiologic confirmation of a biomechanical hypothesis. The American Journal of Sports Medicine. 2019;**47**(1):189-196

[32] Galbusera F, Tornese DZ, Anasetti F, Bersini S, Volpi P, Barbera LL, et al. Does soccer cleat design influence the rotational interaction with the playing surface? Null. 2013;**12**(3):293-301

[33] Jastifer J, Kent R, Crandall J, Sherwood C, Lessley D, McCullough KA, et al. The athletic shoe in football: Apparel or protective equipment? Sports Health. 2017;**9**(2):126-131

[34] Cawley PW, Heidt RS, Scranton PE, Losse GM, Howard ME. Physiologic axial load, frictional resistance, and the football shoe—Surface Interface. Foot & Ankle International. 2003;**24**(7):551-556

[35] Andreasson G, Lindenberger U, Renström P, Peterson L. Torque developed at simulated sliding between sport shoes and an artificial turf. The American Journal of Sports Medicine. 1986;**14**(3):225-230

[36] Takahashi KZ, Gross MT, van Werkhoven H, Piazza SJ, Sawicki GS. Adding stiffness to the foot modulates soleus force-velocity behaviour during human walking. Scientific Reports. 2016;**6**(1):29870

[37] Stefanyshyn DJ, Nigg BM. Influence of midsole bending stiffness on joint energy and jump height performance. Medicine and Science in Sports and Exercise. 2000;**32**(2):471-476

[38] Frimenko RE, Lievers WB, Riley PO, Park JS, Hogan MV, Crandall JR, et al. Development of an injury risk function for first metatarsophalangeal joint sprains. Medicine & Science in Sports & Exercise. 2013;**45**(11):2144-2150

[39] Livesay GA, Reda DR, Nauman EA. Peak torque and rotational stiffness developed at the shoe-surface Interface: The effect of shoe type and playing surface. The American Journal of Sports Medicine. 2006;**34**(3):415-422

[40] Dowling AV, Corazza S, Chaudhari AM, Andriacchi TP. Shoe-surface friction influences movement strategies during a sidestep cutting task: Implications for anterior cruciate ligament injury risk. The American Journal of Sports Medicine. 2010;**38**(3):478-485

[41] Villwock MR, Meyer EG, Powell JW, Fouty AJ, Haut RC. Football playing surface and shoe design affect rotational traction. The American Journal of Sports Medicine. 2009;**37**(3):518-525

[42] Bowers KD Jr, Martin RB. Cleat-surface friction on new and old AstroTurf. Medicine and Science in Sports. 1975;7(2):132-135

[43] Drakos MC, Hillstrom H, Voos JE, Miller AN, Kraszewski AP, Wickiewicz TL, et al. The effect of the shoe-surface Interface in the development of anterior cruciate ligament strain. Journal of Biomechanical Engineering. 2009;**132**(1):011003

[44] Gould HP, Lostetter SJ, Samuelson ER, Guyton GP. Lower extremity injury rates on artificial turf versus natural grass playing surfaces: A systematic review. The American Journal of Sports Medicine. 2022;**50**:3635465211069562

[45] Evolution of the NFL Player | NFL Football Operations. Available at: https://operations.nfl.com/inside-football-ops/players-legends/evolution-of-the-nfl-player/. [Accessed: June 17, 2022]

[46] Wood R. Anthropometry of the Players at the 2018 World Cup. 2018. Available at: https://www.topendsports.com/sport/soccer/anthropometry-worldcup2018.htm. [Accessed: June 17, 2022]

[47] Taylor SA, Fabricant PD, Khair MM, Haleem AM, Drakos MC. A review of synthetic playing surfaces, the shoe-surface interface, and lower extremity injuries in athletes. The Physician and Sportsmedicine. 2012;**40**(4):66-72

[48] Williams S, Hume PA, Kara S. A review of football injuries on third and fourth generation artificial turfs compared with natural turf. Sports Medicine. 2011;**41**(11):903-923

[49] Winson DMG, Miller DLH, Winson IG. Foot injuries, playing surface and shoe design: Should we be thinking more about injury prevention. Foot and Ankle Surgery. 2020;**26**(6):597-600

[50] U.S. Soccer Leagues to Test Out Concussion Substitutes. 2021. Available at: https://www.si.com/soccer/2021/04/05/us-soccer-mls-nwsl-usl-nisa-concussion-substitutes. [Accessed: July 8, 2022]

[51] Goodell: NFL Pledging $100M to Player Safety. 2016. Available at: https://www.espn.com/nfl/story/_/id/17544417/roger-goodell-says-nfl-pledging-100-million-player-safety. [Accessed: Jul 8, 2022]

[52] Moreland G, Barkley LC. Concussion in sport. Current Sports Medicine Reports. 2021;**20**(4):181-182

[53] O'Leary F, Acampora N, Hand F, O'Donovan J. Association of artificial turf and concussion in competitive contact sports: A systematic review and meta-analysis. BMJ Open Sport & Exercise Medicine. 2020;**6**(1):e000695

[54] Meyers MC. Surface-related high school football game injuries on pad and No-pad fields. The American Journal of Sports Medicine. 2021;**49**(9):2489-2497

[55] Guskiewicz KM, Weaver NL, Padua DA, Garrett WE Jr. Epidemiology of concussion in collegiate and high school football players. The American Journal of Sports Medicine. 2000;**28**(5):643-650

[56] Naunheim R, McGurren M, Standeven J, Fucetola R, Lauryssen C, Deibert E. Does the use of artificial turf contribute to head injuries? The Journal of Trauma. 2002;**53**(4):691-694

[57] Heat Levels. Available at: https://www.safehealthyplayingfields.org/heat-levels-synthetic-turf. [Accessed: July 2, 2022]

[58] Williams CF, Pulley GE. Synthetic Turf Heat Studies. Brigham Young University. New Mexico State University College of Agricultural, Consumer, and Environmental Sciences; 2002

[59] Coris EE, Ramirez AM, Van Durme DJ. Heat illness in athletes: The dangerous combination of heat, humidity and exercise. Sports Medicine. 2004;**34**(1):9-16

[60] Seleznow B. Effects of Cold Weather on Artificial Turf Sports Fields. Available at: https://keystonesportsconstruction.com/effects-of-cold-weather-on-artificial-turf-sports-fields/. [Accessed: July 2, 2022]

[61] Knecht E. World cup host Qatar sees climate-controlled stadiums as the future. Reuters. 2019;**26**

[62] Packers' Frozen-Tundra Mystique Melts with Turf-Heating System. 2012. Available at: https://www.nfl.com/news/packers-frozen-tundra-mystique-melts-with-turf-heating-system-09000d5d825faf0a. [Accessed: July 3, 2022]

[63] Sadigursky D, Braid JA, De Lira D, Lemos N, BAB M, RJF C, et al. The FIFA 11+ injury prevention program for soccer players: A systematic review. BMC Sports Science, Medicine and Rehabilitation. 2017;**9**(1):18

[64] Bizzini M, Dvorak J. FIFA 11+: An effective programme to prevent football injuries in various player groups worldwide—A narrative review. British Journal of Sports Medicine. 2015;**49**(9):577

[65] Babault N, Rodot G, Champelovier M, Cometti C. A survey on stretching practices in women and men from various sports or physical activity programs. International Journal of Environmental Research and Public Health. 2021;**18**(8):3928. DOI: 10.3390/ijerph18083928

[66] 2010 NFLPA Playing Surface Opinion Survey. 2011. Available at: www.sportsturfonline.com. [Accessed June 7, 2022]

[67] Most NFL players prefer playing on natural grass. 2009. Available at: www.stma.org. [Accessed: June 5, 2022]

[68] Tretter JC. Only Natural Grass Can Level The NFL's Playing Field. Available at: https://nflpa.com/posts/only-natural-grass-can-level-the-nfls-playing-field. [Accessed: July 5, 2022]

Chapter 4

Injuries in Rugby Union: A Review

Ravin Patel, Austin Wetzler, Nicholas Bennett and Merrick Wetzler

Abstract

Rugby Union is one of the most popular team sports in the world. It is a contact sport that emphasizes possession and control of the ball. By virtue of its full contact nature and lack of protective equipment, Rugby Union is associated with a high incidence of injury relative to many other sports. In fact, Rugby Union carries a significantly higher relative risk of injury than American football, with increase differences in the overall rates of injuries. There are multiple distinct phases of Rugby Union: The Scrum, Tackle, Ruck, Maul and Lineout. Each phase of rugby has its own inherent risk and incidence of injuries which include but not limited to concussions, as well as sprains, strains, and fractures of the upper and lower extremity ligament. The majority of injuries occur either during the scrum and tackling phases of the game. The governing body of Rugby Union is constantly adapting the rules to reduce injuries. Some of these rule changes may have unintended consequences. This article will review the current literature and describe the injuries in each phase of rugby as well as discussing concussion and the effect Covid-19 has had on Rugby Union.

Keywords: rugby, scrum, ruck, maul, tackle, concussion, injuries, cervical spine

1. Introduction

Rugby Union is one of the most popular team sports in the world. It is a contact sport that emphasizes possession and control of the ball. Unlike American football or Rugby League possession of the ball is not necessarily guaranteed after stoppage of play or when the ball carrier is tackled to the ground. It is emphasized with coach and rules to keep the ball in play as much as possible [1, 2].

There are many different forms of the games from touch rugby for the novice players, the seven and ten-man team version, (The seven-man team version is now an Olympic sport), and the classic 15-man version. Each version is based on the same premise that the ball can only be passed backwards, and the goal is for the team to maintain position of the ball and touch the ball down in the try zone. Each version has their own unique incidence of injuries and in this chapter, we will be discussing injuries in the classic 15-man version of Rugby Union [1, 2].

The classic 15-man rugby team (See **Figure 1**) is made up of eight forwards who are usually large and stronger players. There is one Scrumhalf who calls the plays and distributes the ball to the other players and six back line players who do the majority of running and passing the ball. These seven back line players are usually quicker but not as large as the forwards. Rugby Union has multiple discrete phases of play:

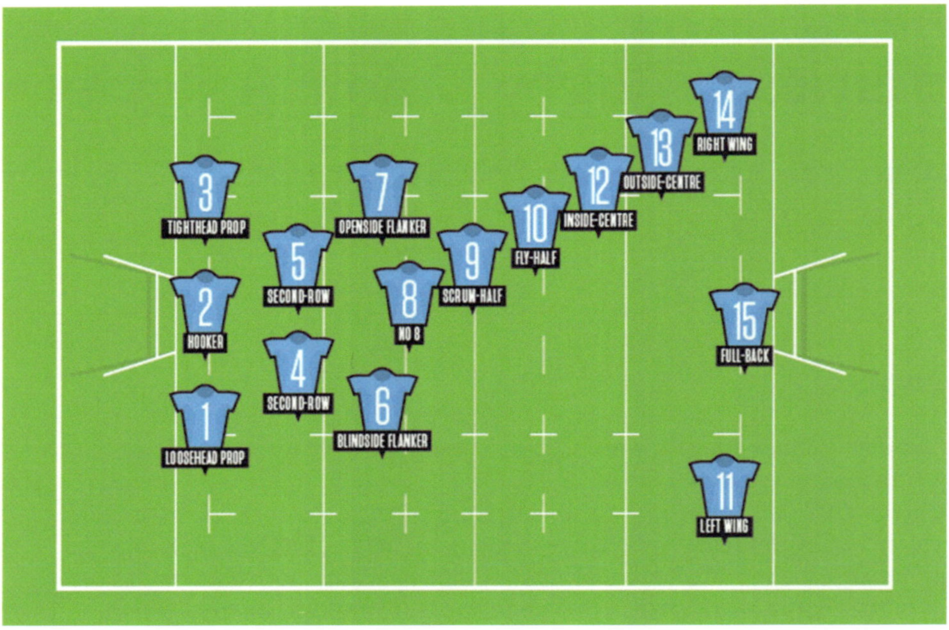

Figure 1.
The 15 players on a Rugby union team (forwards 1–8, scrumhalf 9, backline 10–15).

The scrum, line out, the ruck, the maul, open play, and the tackle. Each phase of the game has its own unique set of injuries with identifiable risk and incidence [1, 2].

The forward or pack players include two props and a hooker, two second rows, two flankers, and one eight men. The players get their names from their position in the pack when a scrum is formed. When a minor infraction occurs to reset play many times a scrum is formed between the two teams to restart play. The front row consists of the hooker and two props the hooker wraps his arms around the props shoulder and the props wrap their inside arm around the hooker's waist holding him (propping) up. Each of the seconds places their head between the hooker and inside arm around the other second rows waist and the outside arm through the legs of the prop and they grab the prop's jersey. The flankers are in the same level as the second row and wrap arms around the second row's waist. Finally, the eight man places his head from behind between the second rows. (See **Figure 2**) [1, 2].

After a minor infraction, the non-penalized team has the opportunity to gain possession and put the ball back into play by rolling the ball in the scrum between the two packs. Each team's pack is assembled with all eight men coming together. Once together, the props touch their opponents' shoulders. After this is done the referee instructs the players to engage through specific commands. Their front rows should engage under control, but one team is always trying to gain the upper hand to control the ball and this interaction in some instances can be quite violent and severe injuries can occur. Once the scrum is formed the hooker signals the scrum half. When the scrumhalf puts the ball between the two packs in the scrum, the hooker uses his/her leg (while being helped up by the props) to sweep the ball towards his side. During this time there can be a lot of jockeying for dominance with pushing and pulling of each scrum which can cause the scrum to rotator or collapse which often result in injuries. The hooker can be very vulnerable because he has his arms around the props

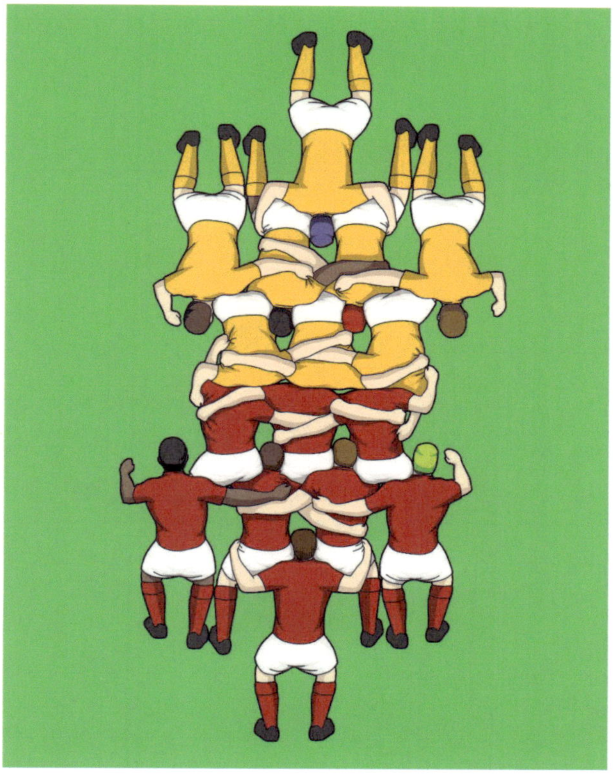

Figure 2.
The two packs of forwards come together to form the scum. Notice how the hooker who is in the front row between the two props arms around them and cannot be used for any mitagation of the forces on engagement of with collapse.

and nothing to protect him if the scrum collapses. The goal of the scrum is to maintain stability and to get the ball to behind the second rows feet where either the eight man or scrum half can take it out of the scrum and restart play [1, 2].

If a ball goes out play the line out is formed and used to restart play. The line out can be made up of part or the entire scrum. The two teams line up a meter apart. The hooker throws the ball in after a play is called. The hooker must throw the ball straight between the two teams. The team throwing the ball in has the advantage of knowing where the ball is being thrown to facilitate restart of play. The players around the one receiving the ball can lift him to allow him to cleanly catch above the opposing players. The player who catches the ball usually tosses the ball or makes it presentable for the scrumhalf to pick it up and toss it to his back line. (See **Figure 3**) [1, 2].

The ruck and mauls are similar and occur after a player is tackled to the ground: The ruck or remains standing: The maul. The goal is to make the ball easily accessible to the scrumhalf to keep the ball in play. Rules have been developed to facilitate presentation of the ball to avoid stoppage of play. (See **Figure 4**) [1, 2].

When a player is tackled the tackling player must wrap their arms around the opponent with the ball. It is a penalty if he strikes the ball carrier without wrapping his arms. The tackler cannot tackle above the shoulders or upper arms (See **Figure 5a**). The tackler is responsible for bringing the player to the ground safely. The tackler cannot lift the player up and forcibly drive the ball carrier to the ground. Once tackled and a ruck

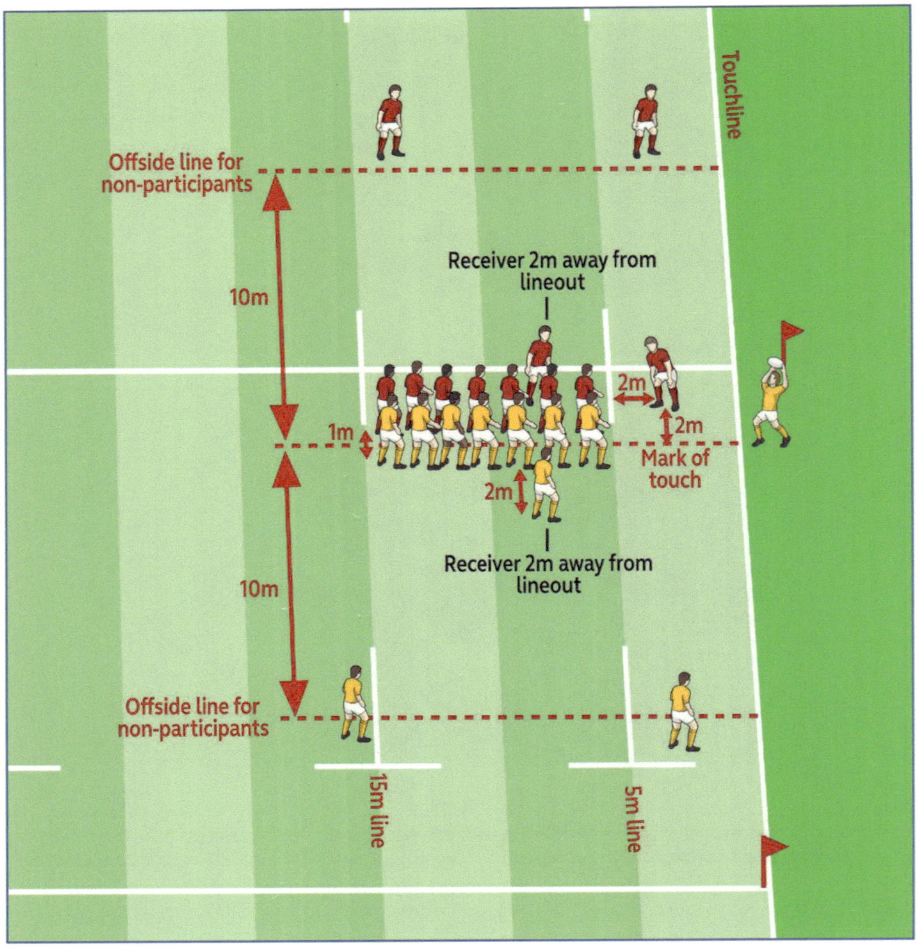

Figure 3.
The lineout. The two lines must be 1 meter apart.

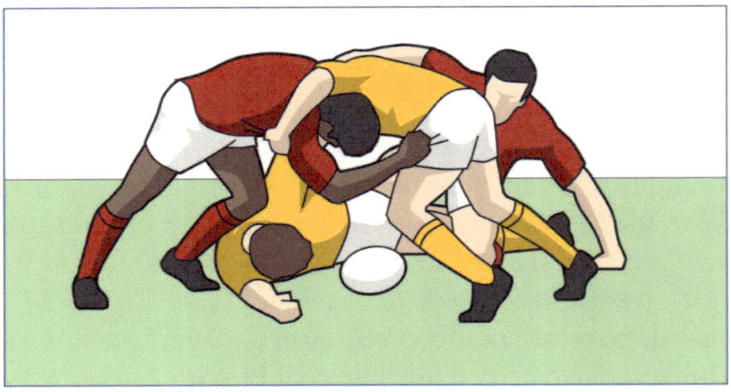

Figure 4.
The ruck is formed after the tackle and one of more players from each team engage which each other.

is formed, the ball carrier must decisively present the ball to be picked up by the scrum half or another available player. If the ball is not presented, then the play is whistled dead, and a scrum is called. The tackler's teammates must stay on their side of tackled ball player, if not they will be called for an offsides penalty [1, 2].

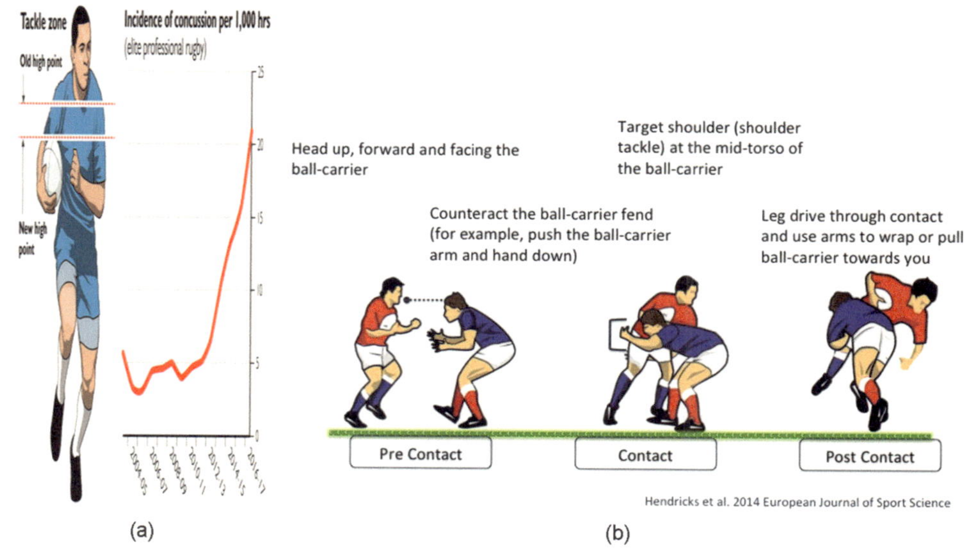

Figure 5.
a: The player must not be tackle above shoulder level. Recent rule changes have lowered as seen in the figure. b: Proper tackling techniques are vitally important to avoid injuries.

The backline players form a line behind the scrumhalf and the ball is tossed backward to them as they run forwards and gain field advantage. In addition to passing the ball backwards, a team can kick the ball forward. When the ball is kicked forwards and remains in the field of play the person who kicked the ball must run and be in front of all his team plays prior to anyone else touching the ball or engaging the player who caught it. Kicking is an important part of rugby but it does not have any incidence of true injuries so it will not be discussed in this article [1, 2].

Each phase of rugby has its own inherent types and incidence of injuries. Most injuries occur during the scrum and tackling phases of the game. The governing body of Rugby Union are constantly adapting to reduce injuries. Major rule changes have been made to make the scrum safer, avoid excessive energy on engagement and avoiding collapse. Additional rules have been made to ensure the ball carrier is tackled safely and given the opportunity to present the ball to his side of the field [1, 2]. Many American football teams teach Rugby Union tackling techniques to reduce the incidence of injury in their players (see **Figure 5b**) [3]. This article will review the current literature and discuss the recent rule changes as applicable.

2. Injuries

By virtue of its full contact nature and lack of protective equipment, rugby is associated with a high incidence of injury relative to many other sports. In fact, a prospective study of collegiate rugby and football demonstrated that rugby carries significantly higher relative risk of injury than football, with pronounced differences in the rates of shoulder, wrist, hand, and lower leg injuries overall [4].

There are several injuries that are an inherent risk of any contact/collision sports such as concussion, upper and lower extremity injury including fractures and ligamentous injuries [5, 6]. Over the past several years there have been procedures and policies put into place to attempt to decrease the incidence of injuries. We have observed similar attempts at this in other sports as well as in American football with tackling policies to reduce the risk of cervical spine and spinal cord injury by avoiding direct contact to the top of the head or helmet by either the tackler or ball carrier [7]. There are additional factors that have been associated with an higher incidence of injury they include games in the earlier part of the season, more veteran and professional high-level matches in a season, and decreased rest for the players between matches [8].

3. Tackle

Rugby Union is distinguished from many sports by the manner in which it combines a quick pace of play with an aggressive, full-contact ruleset [9]. The tackle phase of rugby union occurs more often than any other phase. The tackle phase almost always occurs when at least one player is in motion, usually running at full speed. Many systematic reviews found that the majority of rugby injuries come during the tackle phase of play [10–12]. One study showed that over fifty percent of all rugby union injuries were actually the direct result of tackling or being tackled [10]. Unlike American football, during which players are protected somewhat by a helmet and padding which protects the shoulders, chest, hips, knees, and thighs, rugby players are subjected to several collisions and tackles throughout a match without protective equipment. Studies have shown that the act of tackling, both as the tackler and the tackled, are especially vulnerable for players, as between one third and one half of all rugby injuries occur during the tackle [10–12]. In general, injuries are more common while performing a tackle rather than getting tackled. The tackler is at a higher risk of injury, especially regarding concussion; however, the player being tackled is also at risk of concussion, ligamentous injury, and fracture. A concussion can be either caused by the head hitting the opponent's body, especially in high tackles or when the player goes to the ground and the head can strike the turf. Furthermore, where the ball carrier is tackled there is a different risk of injuries. So, when it comes to the tackle phase, it has been studied that far more injuries occur when the ball carrier is tackled on the middle and high position of the torso. Similarly, it was seen that tackles from the front and side of the individual also result in a higher incidence of injury [10].

There have been some discussions about lowering the level of which the ball carrier can be tackled to below the waist [12]. In the open field this should not be difficult since this is how most tackle occurs anyway. It may fundamentally change the game for the forwards, especially plays off the ruck and back of the scrum where many times a forward would handle the ball and there is only a short distance between him and his opponent. The ability and time to react to the ball carrier would be very limited and could make it difficult to make tackle. Furthermore, this would place the tackler's head nearer to a larger opponent's knee which may increase the chance of concussions. Concussion may also increase as the force the player hits the turf may also be increased. There also may be an increased incidence in ligament injuries of the knee from possible hyperextension or valgus forces placed in the knees during the tackle below the waist [13, 14]. It is agreed that rules changes are necessary as the governing bodies are doing, they are thoroughly venting these changes prior to implementing [1].

As stated previously present, the tackler must wrap and bring the ball carrier safely to the ground. With the changes in the rules allowing the ball carrier to present the ball to his side instead of immediately releasing it, this has kept the ball in play but may have unintended consequences. The senior author who has been involved in both American Football, Rugby Union and Rugby League has observed an increase in the violence of the collision between the ball carrier and tackler. This is especially when the ball carrier is a larger player such as a forward. He sees similarities between Rugby Union and League in the violence of the collision. In Rugby League the player is tackled and held down by their opponent and play is then restarted. Due to rule changes in Rugby Union now, allowing the ball carrier to have increased opportunity to keep the play going after being tackled, the player can go in with increase force. With players now being larger and faster this may cause an increased incidence of significant injuries in the tackling phase of the game, including concussions.

4. Ruck

The ruck is when players are engaged with one another immediately following a tackle. The ruck is formed when at least one player from each team engages over the ball after an attacking player is tackled and subsequently releases the ball. While the tackle is associated with the highest rates of injuries among rugby players, there is also a significant risk of injury during the ruck. Some of the most common injuries that result during the ruck phase are lower extremity ligamentous injuries as players fall onto the legs of their teammates or opponent. Furthermore, lower extremity injuries are most common because of the dynamic nature of participating in a ruck and being upright and the uneven forces that get placed on the lower extremity muscles [4–6, 8]. One study highlighted that that gastrocnemius muscle is often one of the muscles injured during the ruck phase of rugby [6].

5. Scrum

The scrum is a part of the game where players from both teams stand side by side surrounding the ball and come together to ultimately fight for possession of the ball. This constituents of eight players from each team's pack with a total of 16 players involved in the scrum own (See **Figure 1**). The forwards are usually the larger and stronger players [1, 15].

In one study of English scrums, it was found the 31% of the scums were found to result in injury [16]. As with the tackle, devastating catastrophic injury can occur during the scrum and is highly associated with head and spinal cord injury [16–18]. Injuries to the players can happen when they engage their shoulders and neck, the unbalanced forces during the scrum can cause severe damage to an individual's spinal cord if flexed, twisted, or manipulated incorrectly. The scrum can collapse as well, which essentially means the players fold in on one another. The collapsing of the scrum has been shown to have significantly higher rates of injury when compared to scrums that do not collapse. When the scrum collapses, the crown of the head of the props and especially the hooker can strict the ground with significant force resulting in severe cervical spine and or spinal cord injury. The hooker can be especially vulnerable since he cannot protect him or herself when the scrum collapses [16–19].

While many rule changes in rugby over the past decade have centered around reducing the rate of concussions, it is important to highlight other rule changes that have sought to make rugby safer for athletes. The scrum accounts for 40% of spinal injuries sustained by rugby players. Starting in 2013, the pre-scrum sequence was changed to "Crouch, Bind, Set" following a series of alterations over the previous decades. This "bind" command instructed the "props", or the forwards directly engaged with the opposing team during the scrum, to lock onto their opponents prior to the ball being played. This leads to a more stable scrum, but also reduces the multidirectional forces experienced by forwards in the scrum, and thus alters the potential for injuries. Cazzola et al. demonstrated reduced biomechanical loading and c-spine acceleration using the current scrum protocol relative to earlier techniques [20]. Furthermore, this rule change is proposed to decrease the frequency of collapse of the scrum, which has been shown to increase risk for injury in the scrum. Further study will be required to see if this change has led to reductions in injuries from the scrum. There have been rules and regulations to make sure each team has enough skilled players to form and maintain a proper scrum. Additional rules have been made to make under 19-year-old rugby scrums safer and prevent inappropriate cervical loading on these individuals [2].

The scrum can take its toll on a player over the years. It has been shown that individuals participating in the scrum are at risk for both acute spinal cord damage and chronic cervical degeneration. When compared to tackling, the scrum occurs less frequently during the game, however, is associated with a higher risk and relative incidence of injury [16, 18].

6. Lineout

The lineout describes a set piece which occurs after the ball or a player carrying the ball goes outside of the touch line. The line-out then consists of a thrower from one team putting the ball back into play by throwing the ball between groups of players from opposing teams who then lift, or "support" one teammate who goes straight up to receive the thrown ball. This play is associated with lower rates of injuries compared to other phases of play; however, it is often associated with more serious injuries, with one study reporting that 80% of players injured in a line-out were removed from play, which is much higher than other phases of play [9]. Players jumping for the ball are lifted several feet into the air and may be destabilized as they reach for the ball and/or collide with other players. Injuries sustained in lineouts include incarcerated inguinal hernias, ligamentous injuries such as ACL (Anterior Cruciate Ligament) tears, and lumbar and cervical facet injuries [6, 8]. The vulnerable positions created for players, especially those jumping for the ball, has led to restrictions on lineouts for youth rugby players. Typically, full contested lineouts are absent from the game until the U16 level for boys, and U18 for girls. This protects young athletes from the potentially disastrous consequences of lineouts in competitive play [2].

7. Concussion

Concussion is associated with nearly all phases of play during a rugby match or training session. Perhaps not surprisingly, the rate of concussion among rugby players is higher than many other sports with available concussion data. In fact, the rates of concussion are like those seen in boxing. This is primarily due to the intense contact nature of both sports. One literature review looked at the incidence of concussion injury and stratified them specifically by sport. Specifically, concussions accounted for 15% of all injuries experienced by rugby players. This can be further represented when looking at concussion rate per athletic exposure (AE). One systematic review showed the incidence of concussions in match play rugby were a staggering 3/1000 (AE) [13]. This rate is much higher than many other team sports. When comparing American football to collegiate rugby the incidence of injuries is more in rugby. These injuries specifically are concussion and upper extremity ligamentous sprain and strain. Over the past ten to fifteen years, more attention has been brought to the impact of concussions on the game of American football as more is understood about the short- and long-term effects of concussion as well as the additive effects of multiple concussions.

Many concussions that occur in rugby may go underreported as individuals do not want to sit out of play. It has been shown across the board that rugby players actively choose to avoid reporting concussive episodes [21–23]. Analysis of elite level rugby competition have demonstrated that there are a few factors which increase the risk of concussion during a tackle. These factors included acceleration by the tackler into the tackle, high rate of speed of the tackler at time of collision, head-to-head contact, and high tackles. These studies highlighted some of the major challenges in reducing concussions through rule changes implemented in the tackling phase of play [9–12]. For instance, the most obvious rule change that would likely decrease the incidence of concussions in rugby would be to eliminate tackles from the game altogether; however, this change would not be well-received as it would completely change the nature of the game.

Other rule or strategy changes may be more feasible but would have less predictable outcomes on concussion rates. One example of this would be to reduce the amount of space between lines of players on set pieces to reduce the speed of tacklers on these plays. A possible unintended consequence would be that players would likely accelerate into the tackle more frequently given less space to make a play and as stated previously increase ability to keep the ball in play. While increasing enforcement on high tackles and head-to-head contact, the latter of which is already treated with a zero-tolerance policy by World Rugby, may reduce the incidence of these specific types of contact, they may increase the rates of lower tackles and head-to-knee contact, which has also been shown to increase concussion risk.

Over the past several years, there have been many efforts to reduce the rates of concussions in American football competition, including rule changes aimed at reducing head-on collisions involving defenseless players [7]. Perhaps even more important to protecting players have been the advances in reporting and return-to-play protocol. While it is not clear to what extent that the game of rugby has been directly affected by the literature and cultural shifts regarding concussions in American football, there have been changes to the way in which concussions are reported in high-level rugby competition, as well as rule changes aimed to protect players from sequelae of these injuries [1, 2]. Most recently, in June of 2022, World Rugby implemented new changes that lengthened the amount of time players must wait before returning to play after suffering a concussion from seven to twelve days. This change was promoted by the World Rugby independent concussion work group 17-Strong. This rule change will have a large impact on how concussions affect competitive gameplay, as it will in many instances delay players from returning to the subsequent week's competitive play [1].

8. COVID-19

Due to the physical nature of rugby and the proximity of players during various phases of play, additional safety concerns were introduced to the game of rugby during the SARS CoV2 epidemic. Since perhaps the source of the greatest prolonged physical contact comes during the scrum in a rugby match, some leagues reduced or even eliminated the scrum from gameplay during the 2020 season. It is unclear if this measure had any impact on the reduction of Covid 19 transmissions during professional or amateur rugby matches [24, 25]. Furthermore, Jones et al. showed that the risk of transmission of SARS CoV2 was lower than initially predicted, and that in-game transmission could not be confirmed in their study population [26].

9. Summary

Overall, rugby is a physically demanding sport that predisposes individuals to severe injury on occasion. There are several distinct phases of rugby that injury can occur in. It is important to evaluate an individuals' injury in the context of what phase of rugby that the injury occurred in as this can lead to further understanding of the ideology and mechanism of the stated injury. The scrum, ruck and tackling phase of rugby all come with their inherent risks. In the future it would be important to analyze the regulations and rules to utterly understand how to mitigate risk of injury and if rule changes have unintended consequences. Additionally, it is important to maximize players position skill and tackling before entering match play as well as. As with any field sport that requires significant cardiac fitness, optimizing recovery in between matches to ultimately decrease the incidence of injury are important as well. Multiple studies have shown an increase in injuries with fatigue [6, 8].

Author details

Ravin Patel[1], Austin Wetzler[2]*, Nicholas Bennett[3] and Merrick Wetzler[3]

1 Department of Family Practice, Inspira Health Network, Mullica Hill, NJ, USA

2 Lewis Katz School of Medicine, Temple University, Philadelphia, PA, USA

3 Department of Orthopedic Surgery, Philadelphia College of Osteopathic Medicine, Philadelphia, PA, USA

*Address all correspondence to: mjwetz@aol.com

References

[1] World Rugby Union. Available from: https://www.world.rugby

[2] World Rugby – Laws of the game. Available from: www.world.rugby/the-game/laws/home

[3] https://www.nytimes.com/2019/01/02/sports/ncaafootball/football-rugby-texas-tackling-concussions.html?smid=url-share

[4] Willigenburg NW, Borchers JR, Quincy R, Kaeding CC, Hewett TE. Comparison of injuries in American collegiate football and Club Rugby: A prospective cohort study. The American Journal of Sports Medicine. 2016;**44**(3):753-760. DOI: 10.1177/0363546515622389

[5] Williams S, Trewartha G, Kemp S, Stokes K. A meta-analysis of injuries in senior men's professional Rugby union. Sports Medicine. 2013;**43**(10):1043-1055. DOI: 10.1007/s40279-013-0078-1 PMID: 23839770

[6] Yeomans C, Kenny IC, Cahalan R, Warrington GD, Harrison AJ, Hayes K, et al. The incidence of injury in amateur male Rugby union: A systematic review and Meta-analysis. Sports Medicine (Auckland, N.Z.). 2018;**48**(4):837-848. DOI: 10.1007/s40279-017-0838-4

[7] https://www.nytimes.com/2018/09/10/sports/nfl-new-tackling-rule.html

[8] Murias-Lozano R, Mendía L, Sebastián-Obregón FJS, Solís-Mencia C, Hervás-Pérez JP, Garnacho-Castaño MV, et al. The epidemiology of injuries in Spanish Rugby union División de honor. International Journal of Environmental Research and Public Health. 2022;**19**(7):3882. DOI: 10.3390/ijerph19073882 PMID: 35409565; PMCID: PMC8997440

[9] Fuller CW, Brooks JH, Cancea RJ, Hall J, Kemp SP. Contact events in rugby union and their propensity to cause injury. British Journal of Sports Medicine. 2007;**41**(12):862-867. DOI: 10.1136/bjsm.2007.037499\

[10] Edwards S, Lee R, Fuller G, Buchanan M, Tahu T, Tucker R, et al. 3D biomechanics of Rugby tackle techniques to inform future Rugby research practice: A systematic review. Sports Med Open. 2021;7(1):39. DOI: 10.1186/s40798-021-00322-w PMID: 34097146; PMCID: PMC8184906

[11] Gardner AJ, Iverson GL, Williams WH, Baker S, Stanwell P. A systematic review and meta-analysis of concussion in rugby union. Sports Medicine. 2014;**44**(12):1717-1731. DOI: 10.1007/s40279-014-0233-3 PMID: 25138311

[12] Edwards S, Gardner A, Tahu T, Fuller G, Strangman G, Levi CR, et al. Tacklers' head inertial accelerations can Be decreased by altering the way they engage in contact with ball Carriers' torsos. Medicine and Science in Sports and Exercise. 1 Sep 2022;**54**(9):1560-1571. DOI: 10.1249/MSS.0000000000002931 PMID: 35394470

[13] Clay MB, Glover KL, Lowe DT. Epidemiology of concussion in sport: A literature review. Journal of Chiropractic Medicine. 2013;**12**(4):230-251. DOI: 10.1016/j.jcm.2012.11.005

[14] Levy AS, Wetzler MJ, Lewars M, Laughlin W. Knee injuries in women collegiate Rugby players. The

American Journal of Sports Medicine. 1997;**25**:360-362

[15] Bevan T, Chew S, Godsland I, Oliver NS, Hill NE. A game for all shapes and sizes? Changes in anthropometric and performance measures of elite professional rugby union players 1999-2018. BMJ Open Sport & Exercise Medicine. 2022;**8**(1):e001235. DOI: 10.1136/bmjsem-2021-001235 PMID: 35295371; PMCID: PMC8867314

[16] Taylor AE, Kemp S, Trewartha G, Stokes KA. Scrum injury risk in English professional rugby union. British Journal of Sports Medicine. 2014;**48**(13):1066-1068. DOI: 10.1136/bjsports-2013-092873

[17] Wetzler MJ, Akpata T, Albert T, Foster TE, Levy AS. A retrospective study of cervical spine injuries in American Rugby, 1970 to 1994. The American Journal of Sports Medicine. 1996;**24**(4):454-458. DOI: 10.1177/036354659602400408

[18] Wetzler MJ, Akpata T, Laughlin W, Levy AS. Occurrence of cervical spine injuries during the Rugby scrum. The American Journal of Sports Medicine. 1998;**26**(2):177-180. DOI: 10.1177/03635465980260020501

[19] Milburn PD. Biomechanics of rugby union scrummaging. Technical and safety issues. Sports medicine (Auckland, N.Z.). 1993;**16**(3):168-179. DOI: 10.2165/00007256-199316030-00002

[20] Cazzola D, Stone B, Holsgrove TP, Trewartha G, Preatoni E. Spinal muscle activity in simulated rugby union scrummaging is affected by different engagement conditions. Scandinavian Journal of Medicine & Science in Sports. 2016;**26**(4):432-440. DOI: 10.1111/sms.12446 PMID: 25818526

[21] McCrory P, Feddermann-Demont N, Dvořák J, Cassidy JD, McIntosh A, Vos PE, et al. What is the definition of sports-related concussion: A systematic review. British Journal of Sports Medicine. 2017;**51**(11):877-887. DOI: 10.1136/bjsports-2016-097393

[22] Longworth T, McDonald A, Cunningham C, Khan H, Fitzpatrick J. Do rugby league players under-report concussion symptoms? A cross-sectional study of elite teams based in Australia. BMJ Open Sport & Exercise Medicine. 2021;**7**(1):e000860. DOI: 10.1136/bmjsem-2020-000860 PMID: 33520253; PMCID: PMC7817803

[23] Musumeci G, Ravalli S, Amorini AM, Lazzarino G. Concussion in sports. Journal of functional morphology and kinesiology. 2019;**4**(2):37. DOI: 10.3390/jfmk4020037

[24] Sewry N, Schwellnus M, Readhead C, Swanevelder S, Jordaan E. The incidence and transmission of SARS-CoV-2 infection in south African professional rugby players - AWARE II. Journal of Science and Medicine in Sport. 2022;**25**(8):639-643. DOI: 10.1016/j.jsams.2022.06.004 PMID: 35791997; PMCID: PMC9197565

[25] Stokes KA, Jones B, Bennett M, Close GL, Gill N, Hull JH, et al. Returning to play after prolonged training restrictions in professional collision sports. International Journal of Sports Medicine. 2020;**41**(13):895-911. DOI: 10.1055/a-1180-3692 PMID: 32483768; PMCID: PMC7799169

[26] Jones B, Phillips G, Kemp S, Payne B, Hart B, Cross M, et al. SARS-CoV-2 transmission during rugby league matches: Do players become infected after participating with SARS-CoV-2 positive players? British Journal of Sports Medicine. 2021;**55**(14):807-813. DOI: 10.1136/bjsports-2020-103714 PMID: 33574043; PMCID: PMC7886661

Chapter 5

Lisfranc Injury in the Athlete

Austin Lee, Philip Shaheen, Christopher Kreulen and Eric Giza

Abstract

Lisfranc injuries refer to a disruption or destabilization of the Lisfranc joint complex or tarsometatarsal joint complex. These injuries are relatively rare; however, clinical signs are subtle with the injury diagnosis frequently missed. A delay in diagnosis can negatively impact the patient's outcome with sequelae ranging from post-traumatic osteoarthritis to a dysfunctional foot. Therefore, evaluating midfoot injuries requires a high index of suspicion and thorough examination for a tarsometatarsal joint complex injury to allow for maximal return of function and rapid return to sport. The mechanism of Lisfranc injuries in athletes tend to be relatively low-energy which differs from more common higher-energy injuries such as car accidents. Most importantly, identifying and treating Lisfranc injuries requires understanding of the structural anatomy and stability of the midfoot.

Keywords: lisfranc, midfoot, athlete, sports, tarsometatarsal

1. Introduction

The tarsometatarsal (TMT) joint complex is also known as the Lisfranc joint complex. The Lisfranc joint complex is named after one of Napoleon Bonaparte's field surgeons, Jacques Lisfranc, who described cavalry officer injuries and amputations for gangrene through this joint [1]. Thus, a Lisfranc injury refers to a disruption or destabilization of the bones and/or ligaments constructing the TMT joint complex. These injuries are relatively uncommon, occurring in 1 per 55,000 people yearly, which comprises around 0.2% of all fractures [2]. However on initial evaluation, up to 20% of Lisfranc injuries are estimated to be misdiagnosed or completely missed [3]. A delay in diagnosis can negatively impact the patient's outcome and recovery with sequelae ranging from post-traumatic osteoarthritis to a permanently dysfunctional foot [4]. In athletes, these injuries can prohibit players from sport and potentially hinder them from returning to the same level of performance after recovery. Therefore, evaluating midfoot injuries requires a high index of suspicion and thorough examination for a TMT joint complex injury to allow for maximal return of function and rapid return for athletes to sport.

In this chapter, we will discuss evaluation and workup for Lisfranc injuries as well as non-operative and operative treatment of Lisfranc injuries with its impact on athletes.

2. Anatomy

The Lisfranc joint complex refers to the bony and ligamentous midfoot complex comprised of the cuboid and medial, middle, and lateral cuneiform articulating with the five metatarsal bones [1]. The structure's transverse arch resembles the renowned architectural Roman arch, with the second TMT joint serving as the keystone. This bony organization ultimately provides structural stability like the Roman arch to prevent plantar displacement when load bearing on the foot [5].

There are three longitudinal columns that organize the Lisfranc joint complex: the medial, middle, and lateral columns. The medial column consists of the first metatarsal and navicular-medial cuneiform articulation, and the middle column consists of the second and third metatarsal articulating with the middle and lateral cuneiforms [6]. The lateral column consists of the fourth and fifth metatarsal articulating with the cuboid, middle cuneiform, and lateral cuneiform [7].

The TMT ligaments on the dorsal and plantar aspects stabilize the TMT joints, with the second through fifth metatarsals having both dorsal and plantar intermetatarsal ligaments providing stability between these bones [6]. The first and second metatarsals do not have an intermetatarsal ligament, instead having a dorsal, interosseous, and plantar ligaments bridging the medial cuneiform to the second metatarsal [1, 7]. The interosseous ligament is also known as the Lisfranc ligament and serves as the strongest ligamentous stabilizer between the medial cuneiform and second metatarsal [2]. The dorsal ligament is 4.5 times smaller than the plantar ligament and commonly believed to be the weakest ligament of the complex [7].

In addition to the bony and ligamentous architecture of the Lisfranc joint complex, neurovascular structures and muscle tendons are in close-proximity and important to consider when evaluating and operating on a Lisfranc injury. Between the base of the first and second metatarsals, the dorsalis pedis artery and deep peroneal nerve travel on the dorsal aspect of the foot [8]. If there is dorsal displacement with a Lisfranc injury, these structures could be damaged. The anterior tibial tendon is found attaching to the medial cuneiform and base of the first metatarsal, while the peroneus brevis is found attaching to the base of the fifth metatarsal [2]. These structures can potentially block and prevent injury reduction depending on the injury pattern.

3. Mechanism of injury

In the general population, Lisfranc injuries most frequently occur in higher-energy trauma such as car crashes; however, lower energy-impacts are more commonly the cause of Lisfranc injuries in athletes [9]. These injuries may involve bone fractures or be purely ligamentous. In athletes, injury to the TMT joint complex typically results indirectly when a plantar flexed foot loaded axially with or without rotation causes hyper plantar flexion of the forefoot [10], subsequently causing the dorsal ligaments to rupture. On the plantar surface, the plantar capsule may rupture, or the base of the metatarsal may fracture, resulting in midfoot instability from free movement of the metatarsals dorsally [11]. For example, this injury can occur in an athlete falling onto a plantar flexed foot or in an athlete making a sudden change in direction (i.e. rotation) on a plantar flexed foot. These injuries can also occur from direct forces to the athlete such as a direct crushing force on the midfoot.

4. Diagnosis

TMT joint complex injuries can range from a mild subluxation to fracture-dislocations; thus, patients can present with a variety of symptoms. Most consistently, an injury to the TMT joint complex presents with weight-bearing midfoot pain, which can also be induced by testing the joint with passive pronation-abduction [12]. Another potential sign indicating a Lisfranc injury is midfoot swelling [10]. Plantar ecchymosis of the foot arch suggests soft tissue disruption and should greatly increase the index of suspicion for a Lisfranc injury [13]. A 'positive gap' refers to an increased distance between the hallux and second toe which indicates increased intercuneiform instability and can indicate a Lisfranc injury [4]. Additionally, athletes will typically describe a 'pop' in the foot directly preceding a Lisfranc injury, but this history is not necessary to diagnose an injury to the TMT joint complex [14]. Clinical signs and symptoms combined with an appropriate history and mechanism of the patient's injury warrants further workup and evaluation for a Lisfranc injury.

When there is clinical suspicion of a Lisfranc injury, an initial set of AP, lateral, and oblique X-Rays of the foot should be obtained to visualize the TMT joint. Ideally weight-bearing x-rays are taken because the stress can reveal intra-articular diastasis that can self-reduce when the stress of weight bearing is removed. In Nunley and Vertullo's study establishing their classification system for Lisfranc injuries, half of the athletes with midfoot injuries had normal non-weightbearing imaging [15]. Unfortunately the initial set of injury radiographs are often not weight bearing due to pain in the acute post-injury setting precluding weight bearing on the injured foot. Regardless, there is still utility in assessing non weight bearing x-rays for subtle signs of injury, particularly when they are paired with an x-ray of the contralateral, non-injured foot for comparison. When examining an AP view of a normal midfoot, the medial base of the second metatarsal should align with the medial border of the intermediate cuneiform. In addition, there should be symmetric joint spaces along the medial longitudinal column, particularly at the articulation of the medial column and the base of the second metatarsal. On an oblique view, the medial base of the third metatarsal should align with the medial border of the lateral cuneiform in the absence of injury. If there are any step-offs in these lines, then a Lisfranc injury should be suspected. Radiographic findings of dorsal displacement of the metatarsals, >2 mm diastasis of the space between the first metatarsal-medial cuneiform and second metatarsal when compared to the contralateral side, or > 2 mm of TMT joint subluxation indicate instability to the Lisfranc joint [16]. A small avulsion fracture of the second metatarsal base known as the "fleck sign" suggests a Lisfranc ligament avulsion injury [11].

For subtle injuries where a Lisfranc injury is still suspected given appropriate history, mechanism of injury, signs, and symptoms, a weight bearing AP view of both feet on the same cassette or an AP pronation-abduction stress radiograph can help identify dynamic instability by stressing the tarsometatarsal joint complex (**Figure 1**) [16]. Weight-bearing on a Lisfranc injury can be a very painful experience for the patient. Therefore, it is important to inform the patient the reason for obtaining a weight bearing radiograph, since the pain can inadvertently result in uneven weight distribution across the patient's feet and a falsely negative result [17]. Because of major patient discomfort, these radiographs can be obtained using a nerve block or general anesthesia, but this is rarely performed [16, 17].

Advanced imaging modalities such as computed tomography are helpful after inconclusive initial imaging to evaluate subtle fracture-comminution and subluxations. CT scans can also help with surgical planning to decide between primary

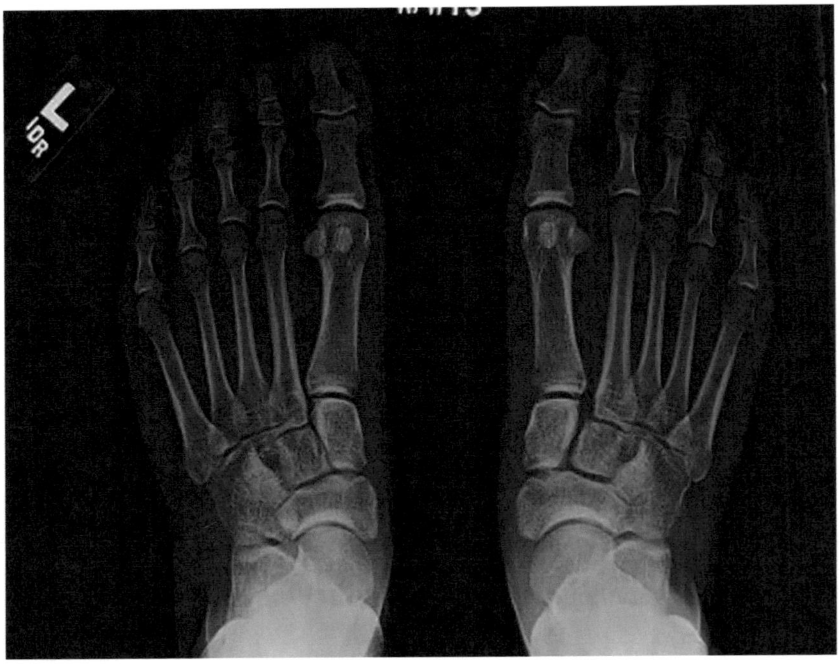

Figure 1.
Bilateral AP X-ray of the feet showing > 2 mm diastasis between the right first metatarsal-medial cuneiform and second metatarsal.

arthrodesis versus open reduction with internal fixation [4]. One pitfall of CT is its static nature without weight bearing which limits its capabilities to help evaluate dynamic stability [9]. Weight bearing CT scan is a newer modality that aims to correct some of the deficiencies of CT scans but these not yet widespread and may be of limited utility in the initial post-injury phase due to pain limiting the patients ability to weight. Magnetic resonance imaging is useful to evaluate subtle soft tissue damage in purely ligamentous injuries and stability of the Lisfranc joint, which is a particularly useful tool in athletes where ligamentous Lisfranc injuries are more frequent compared to the general population [14]. When detecting a plantar Lisfranc ligament injury, an MRI exhibited a 95% sensitivity, 75% specificity, and 94% positive predictive value [18].

5. Classification

There are two leading classification systems for categorizing Lisfranc injuries: the Myerson and Nunley-Vertullo systems [9, 19].

The Myerson classification system is commonly used to provide a standardized approach towards describing high-grade Lisfranc injuries (**Table 1**) [19, 20]. In 1909, Quenu and Kuss created the first Lisfranc injury classification system which was modified in 1982 by Hardcastle et al. [13] to describe three patterns: type A or total incongruity, type B or partial incongruity, and type C or divergent [20]. The Myerson classification system further modified the Hardcastle system in 1986, and divided type B and C into types B1, B2, C1, and C2. Type B1 specifies partial incongruity with medial displacement, while type B2 specifies partial incongruity with lateral

Myerson	Type description	Nunley-vertullo	Stage description
Type A	Total incongruity	Stage I	No displacement with positive bone scan
Type B1	Partial incongruity with medial displacement	Stage II	Diastasis without a loss in arch height
Type B2	Partial incongruity with lateral displacement		
Type C1	Divergent pattern with partial displacement	Stage III	Diastasis with a loss in arch height
Type C2	Divergent pattern with total displacement		

Table 1.
Comparison of the Myerson classification system typing and Nunley-Vertullo classification system staging.

displacement. Type C1 specifies a divergent pattern with partial displacement, while type C2 specifies a divergent pattern with total displacement [20, 21]. It is important to note that the Myerson classification system is simply a descriptive tool and does not translate to predicting prognosis or determining direct decisions for treatment [13].

The Nunley-Vertullo classification system is advantageous when compared to the Myerson system in its ability to describe low-grade Lisfranc injuries in athletes (**Table 1**) [19]. In addition to its usefulness in athletes, this classification system aids in clinical management by staging the injury and recommending non-operative versus operative treatment depending on the stage. Stage I describes a nondisplaced midfoot with a positive bone scan, which is the only stage that is recommended to be treated non-operatively. Stage II describes diastasis without a loss in arch height, and stage III describes diastasis with a loss in arch height. Injuries graded stage II or III warrant operative management [15]. When it is unclear if a Lisfranc injury is a Nunley-Vertullo Stage I versus Stage II, an MRI can help evaluate the Lisfranc ligament to determine the stage and subsequent treatment plan [22].

6. Treatment

6.1 Non-operative

In patients where there is no evidence of displacement, diastasis, or instability on weightbearing radiographs, their Lisfranc injury is stable [11]. These patients are classified as Stage I using the Nunley-Vertullo classification system and can properly be managed non-operatively [15]. A short-leg cast or a walker boot with protected weightbearing as tolerable for 4–6 weeks is the initial treatment, and weight-bearing radiographs 2 weeks from the injury should be obtained to ensure there is no displacement [6, 17]. If pain persists, a walker boot with weight-bearing permitted can be used for an additional 4 weeks [4, 13]. Stage I Lisfranc injuries can take patients anywhere from 8 to 16 weeks to recover [11]. Despite athletes having to spend a couple of months away from sport, Nunley and Vertullo report that there is a 93% patient satisfaction with this treatment [15]. Therefore, it is important to inform athletes of the recovery timeframe and patient satisfaction at the beginning of treatment before they can return to sport to ensure treatment adherence.

6.2 Operative

Stage II and stage III Lisfranc injuries are unstable and require operative management to achieve reduction [15]. In instances of severe dislocations or compartment syndrome, the injury should be quickly addressed to prevent further complications via reduction or compartment release, respectively [11]. Otherwise, surgical intervention should be delayed 10 to 14 days to allow the soft tissue to heal [4, 16].

In predominantly ligamentous injuries, interosseous transarticular solid screw fixation is thought to be best at holding a reduction to allow the ligament to heal [11]. There is debate whether primary arthrodesis or open reduction with internal fixation (ORIF) yields better results long term for patients with primarily or purely ligamentous Lisfranc injuries in terms of maintaining reduction, degree of deformity, and rate of re-operations [23, 24]. Some surgeons prefer ORIF as a primary treatment choice with primary arthrodesis reserved as a salvage procedure, in cases of late presentation, or in cases of severe articular damage [6, 11]. However, Ly and Coetzee found in a randomized clinical trial that primary arthrodesis has better short and medium-term outcomes than ORIF in primarily ligamentous injuries [25]. It should be noted that ORIF may require a greater reoperation rate when compared to primary arthrodesis, and some studies suggest that there is no statistically significant difference in physical functioning between the two surgeries [23, 24, 26]. With either approach, achieving anatomical reduction and stable fixation should be the ultimate goal [6, 9, 11, 23, 24]. Reduction can be defined as a < 2 mm intercuneiform distance, $<15^{\circ}$ TMT angle, and absent metatarsal displacement in the dorsal or plantar planes [5]. In the athlete population, it is important to consider athletic performance and restoring midfoot stability; there may be some exceptions in young highly active athletes where ORIF might be considered over primary arthrodesis [13]. These authors prefer ORIF as an operative treatment for athletes.

6.3 Post-operative

Post-operative management for ORIF and primary arthrodesis are the same with non-weightbearing for 6 weeks after surgery, suture removal 2 to 3 weeks post-operation, short-leg cast or boot for 3 to 4 weeks, then weightbearing with arch support insert in a boot, and eventual transition to normal shoes 3 months after the operation [2, 11]. In high performing athletes, pool therapy can be initiated after wounds have healed, and after 4 weeks, stationary bike without resistance can be started [11]. At 12 weeks, running with modified shoes is allowed without cutting or sprinting for another month, then the athlete can gradually return to sport [11]. Screws and plates except inter-cuneiform screws for proximal or medial column injuries after ORIF are removed 4 to 6 months after surgery if there is no radiographic evidence of remaining instability, and athletes should avoid contact sports for 6 to 8 weeks after hardware removal [11, 14].

Regardless of reduction and fixation choice, recovery from Lisfranc injuries largely depends on the degree of instability at the TMT joint [12]. Furthermore, the most common complication from a Lisfranc injury is post-traumatic arthritis which depends on the quality of reduction and amount of articular damage present [24]. A majority of athletes will be able to return to sports after a period of recovery and rehabilitation [27–29], with athletes sustaining ligamentous injuries able to return to sport quicker on average than those with bony injuries [28]. It should be noted that athletes may have deep peroneal nerve sensation loss [28], and athletic level of performance usually decreases after returning from injury [29]. Therefore, it is important to inform athletes of all levels that they may not be able to return to high-level sports, and their level of performance can be affected after recovering from a Lisfranc injury.

7. Surgical technique

7.1 Exposure and reduction

After general anesthesia induction, C-arm fluoroscopy is used to examine and demonstrate instability and opening at the Lisfranc joint with foot manipulation when compared to the contralateral side.

After prepping and draping the foot and ankle in a sterile fashion, a 2-4 cm incision is made just laterally to the second metatarsal's lateral border. Fluoroscopy should be used to mark the incision, since being too medial over the second metatarsal shaft is a common mistake. This makes it difficult to work on the metatarsal's lateral border without causing soft tissue stretching or extending the incision. Scissor dissection is carefully performed down to bone with electrocautery to achieve hemostasis. Care is taken to protect any superficial peroneal nerve branches, and the extensor hallucis brevis is bluntly retracted medially to protect the neurovascular bundle.

The soft tissues are elevated from lateral to medial towards the Lisfranc region, where a portion of the dorsal Lisfranc ligament may be visualized running obliquely from the medial cuneiform to the second metatarsal. These oblique fibers may be homogenous and lacking direction in a scarred, chronic injury or disrupted in an acute tear. A Freer elevator is placed in the Lisfranc's articulation and confirmed with fluoroscopy (**Figure 2**). In the instance of a tear, the Freer will pass easily, but it will not normally pass between the medial cuneiform and second metatarsal. Likewise, intercuneiform disruption can be assessed since the freer should not be able to pass between the medial and intermediate cuneiforms. In the presence of intercuneiform instability, a bridge plating construct can address this issue separately. After an isolated ligamentous Lisfranc injury is confirmed, debris is removed from the joint, and any bridge plating for TMT subluxations can be performed.

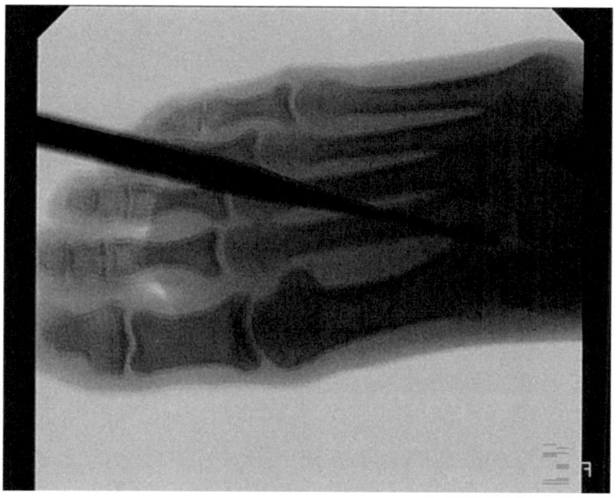

Figure 2.
X-ray of a freer elevator in the Lisfranc articulation.

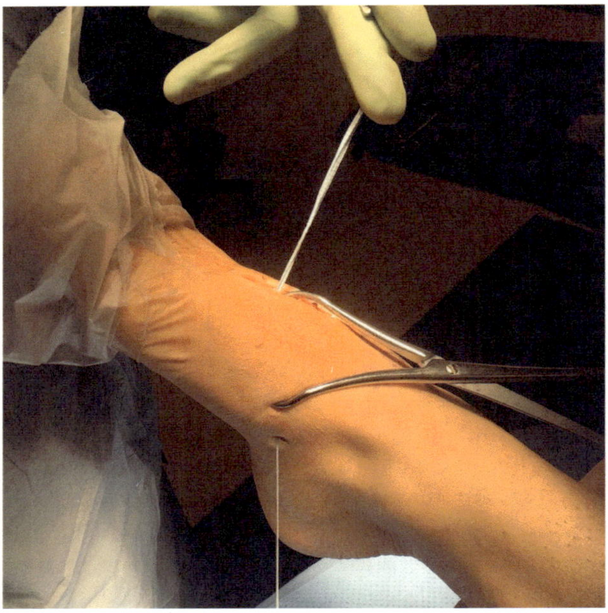

Figure 3.
Lisfranc joint reduction using a large clamp.

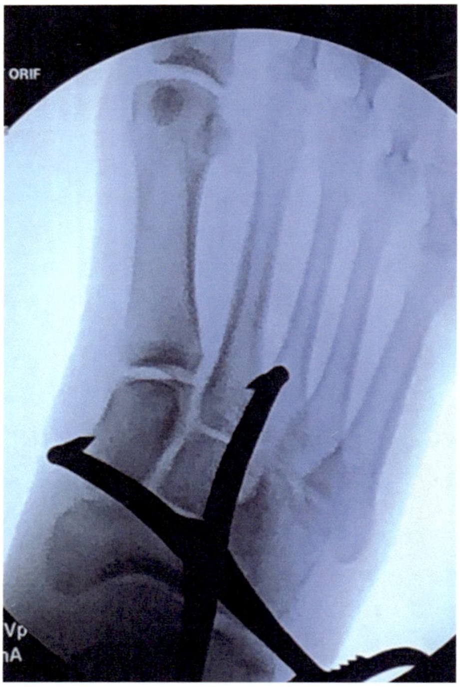

Figure 4.
Fluoroscopic confirmation for the Lisfranc joint reduction.

At the border of the medial cuneiform, a percutaneous incision is made. The joint is reduced with a large clamp towards the Lisfranc joint (**Figure 3**) and confirmed using fluoroscopy (**Figure 4**). The TMT joints are evaluated to ensure that joint subluxation was not caused by the clamping.

7.2 Lisfranc repair with *Internal Brace*

Laterally at second metatarsal base just distal to the articulation with the third metatarsal base, a 1.6 mm specialized passing wire is placed. Under fluoroscopic guidance in line with the Lisfranc ligament trajectory, the wire is advanced through the second metatarsal base into the medial cuneiform. The wire's ideal exit point from the medial cuneiform is at the middle from dorsal to plantar, at or just proximal to the bony protuberance often seen on the medial aspect, and plantar and proximal to the obliquely crossing tibialis anterior tendon medially. The wire is continued to be advanced through the medial cuneiform to the medial skin, and a 1–2 cm incision is made to let the wire pass.

A 3.5 mm cannulated drill is placed over the medial portion of the wire to drill approximately 18 mm into the medial cuneiform for the interference screw, with fluoroscopy to confirm that the drill did not violate the medial cuneiform's lateral cortex. If the bone quality is outstanding, the wire is pulled back and a 4.75 mm tap is advanced into the cuneiform approximately 7 mm.

The FiberTape is threaded through a small stainless steel button, then using a passing wire, the 2 mm FiberTape-button construct is passed from lateral to medial. When passing the FiberTape and wire through the bone tunnel, it is important to use the drill's oscillate function. Afterwards, ensure that there is excellent apposition of the small button at the lateral second metatarsal. Pull tightly while diverging the suture limbs away from each other, place a 4.75 × 15 mm PEEK interference screw between the limbs, and advance until the end of the screw is level with the medial cortex.

The clamp is removed, and stability is confirmed under direct visualization by stressing the joint (**Figure 5**). It should no longer be possible to pass a freer into the

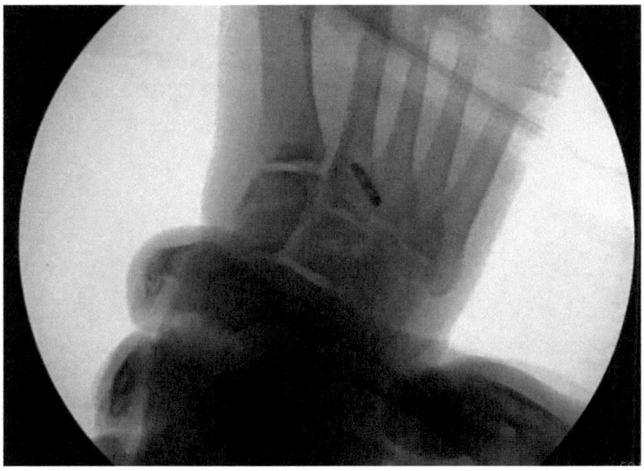

Figure 5.
Confirmation of Lisfranc joint stability under stress.

joint. Fluoroscopy can also be used to confirm the reduction and stability with stress. After irrigating the wound, the incision is closed, and a splint is applied.

Post-operatively, patients are initially kept non-weight bearing with gradual progression of weight bearing sometimes being initiated in the 4–6 week postop period and weight bearing as tolerated often being permitted in the 8–12 week postop timeframe.

8. Conclusion

Lisfranc injuries are relatively uncommon when compared to the frequency of all fractures, but its potentially subtle presentation and severe consequences if missed should make clinicians suspect this injury in patients who present with midfoot trauma [16]. Proper imaging workup with a high index of suspicion is imperative to detect injuries to the TMT joint given the frequency these injuries are misdiagnosed or missed [3]. Stable Nunley Vertullo Stage I Lisfranc injuries can be treated nonoperatively with excellent outcomes, but athletes should be informed of the timeframe for recovery [15]. Unstable Nunley Vertullo Stage II and Stage III Lisfranc injuries should be treated aggressively with ORIF or primary arthrodesis [15]. Understanding the anatomy of the TMT joint complex is essential in operatively treating and stabilizing Lisfranc injuries. For athletes, it is imperative to be honest about treatment outcomes, recovery timeframe, and realistic expected level of play to manage expectations.

Author details

Austin Lee, Philip Shaheen*, Christopher Kreulen and Eric Giza
UC Davis Health System, Sacramento, CA, USA

*Address all correspondence to: philipjshaheen@gmail.com

References

[1] de Palma L, Santucci A, Sabetta SP, Rapali S. Anatomy of the Lisfranc joint complex. Foot & Ankle International. 1997;**18**(6):356-364

[2] Desmond EA, Chou LB. Current concepts review: Lisfranc injuries. Foot & Ankle International. 2006;**27**(8):653-660

[3] Trevino SG, Kodros S. Controversies in tarsometatarsal injuries. The Orthopedic Clinics of North America. 1995;**26**(2):229-238

[4] Moracia-Ochagavía I, Rodríguez-Merchán EC. Lisfranc fracture-dislocations: current management. EFORT Open Reviews. 2019;**4**(7):430-444

[5] Lee CA, Birkedal JP, Dickerson EA, Vieta PA Jr, Webb LX, Teasdall RD. Stabilization of Lisfranc joint injuries: A biomechanical study. Foot & Ankle International. 2004;**25**(5):365-370

[6] Clare MP. Lisfranc injuries. Current Reviews in Musculoskeletal Medicine. 2017;**10**(1):81-85

[7] Johnson A, Hill K, Ward J, Ficke J. Anatomy of the lisfranc ligament. Foot & Ankle Specialist. 2008;**1**(1):19-23

[8] Chitra R. The relationship between the deep fibular nerve and the dorsalis pedis artery and its surgical importance. Indian Journal of Plastic Surgery. 2009;**42**(1):18-21

[9] DeOrio M, Erickson M, Usuelli FG, Easley M. Lisfranc injuries in sport. Foot and Ankle Clinics. 2009;**14**(2):169-186

[10] Shapiro MS, Wascher DC, Finerman GA. Rupture of Lisfranc's ligament in athletes. The American Journal of Sports Medicine. 1994;**22**(5): 687-691

[11] Lewis JS Jr, Anderson RB. Lisfranc injuries in the athlete. Foot & Ankle International. 2016;**37**(12):1374-1380

[12] Curtis MJ, Myerson M, Szura B. Tarsometatarsal joint injuries in the athlete. The American Journal of Sports Medicine. 1993;**21**(4):497-502

[13] Grewal US, Onubogu K, Southgate C, Dhinsa BS. Lisfranc injury: A review and simplified treatment algorithm. Foot (Edinburgh, Scotland). 2020;**45**:101719

[14] Anderson RB, Hunt KJ, McCormick JJ. Management of common sports-related injuries about the foot and ankle. American Academy of Orthopaedic Surgeon. 2010;**18**(9):546-556

[15] Nunley JA, Vertullo CJ. Classification, investigation, and management of midfoot sprains: Lisfranc injuries in the athlete. The American Journal of Sports Medicine. 2002;**30**(6):871-878

[16] Weatherford BM, Anderson JG, Bohay DR. FACS management of tarsometatarsal joint injuries. Journal of the American Academy of Orthopaedic Surgeons. 2017;**25**(7):469-479

[17] Watson TS, Shurnas PS, Denker J. Treatment of Lisfranc joint injury: Current concepts. American Academy of Orthopaedic Surgeon. 2010;**18**(12):718-728

[18] Raikin SM, Elias I, Dheer S, Besser MP, Morrison WB, Zoga AC. Prediction of midfoot instability in the subtle Lisfranc injury. Comparison of magnetic resonance imaging with

intraoperative findings. The Journal of Bone and Joint Surgery. American Volume. 2009;**91**(4):892-899

[19] Chung JH, Mark S, Boyle DE. Classification, diagnosis, and treatment of Lisfranc injuries: A systematic qualitative review. Polymyalgia Rheumatica. 2014;**15**(19):15-27

[20] Mahmoud S, Hamad F, Riaz M, Ahmed G, Al Ateeq M, Ibrahim T. Reliability of the Lisfranc injury radiological classification (Myerson-modified Hardcastle classification system). International Orthopaedics. 2015;**39**(11):2215-2218. DOI: 10.1007/s00264-015-2939-8

[21] Myerson MS, Fisher RT, Burgess AR, Kenzora JE. Fracture dislocations at the tarsometatarsal joints: End results correlated with pathology and treatment. Foot & Ankle. 1986;**6**:225-242

[22] Thevendran G, Kadakia AR, Giza E, et al. Acute foot and ankle injuries and time return to sport. SICOT Journal. 2021;7:27. DOI: 10.1051/sicotj/2021024

[23] Henning JA, Jones CB, Sietsema DL, Bohay DR, Anderson JG. Open reduction internal fixation versus primary arthrodesis for Lisfranc injuries: A prospective randomized study. Foot & Ankle International. 2009;**30**(10):913-922. DOI: 10.3113/FAI.2009.0913

[24] Smith N, Stone C, Furey A. Does open reduction and internal fixation versus primary arthrodesis improve patient outcomes for Lisfranc trauma? A systematic review and Meta-analysis. Clinical Orthopaedics and Related Research. 2016;**474**(6):1445-1452. DOI: 10.1007/s11999-015-4366-y

[25] Ly TV, Coetzee JC. Treatment of primarily ligamentous Lisfranc joint injuries: Primary arthrodesis compared with open reduction and internal fixation. A prospective, randomized study. The Journal of Bone and Joint Surgery. American Volume. 2006;**88**(3):514-520. DOI: 10.2106/JBJS.E.00228

[26] Kuo RS, Tejwani NC, Digiovanni CW, et al. Outcome after open reduction and internal fixation of Lisfranc joint injuries. The Journal of Bone and Joint Surgery. American Volume. 2000;**82**(11):1609-1618. DOI: 10.2106/00004623-200011000-00015

[27] MacMahon A, Kim P, Levine DS, et al. Return to sports and physical activities after primary partial arthrodesis for Lisfranc injuries in young patients. Foot & Ankle International. 2016;**37**(4):355-362

[28] Deol RS, Roche A, Calder JD. Return to training and playing after acute Lisfranc injuries in elite professional soccer and Rugby players. The American Journal of Sports Medicine. 2016;**44**(1):166-170

[29] McHale KJ, Rozell JC, Milby AH, Carey JL, Sennett BJ. Outcomes of Lisfranc injuries in the National Football League. The American Journal of Sports Medicine. 2016;**44**(7):1810-1817. DOI: 10.1177/0363546516645082